Community-Oriented Primary Care: Health Care for the 21st century

Edited by
Robert Rhyne, M.D., Richard Bogue, Ph.D.,
Gary Kukulka, Ph.D., Hugh Fulmer, M.D.

D0878729

American Public Health Association
1015 Fifteenth Street, NW
Washington, DC 20005

Community-Oriented Primary Care:
Health Care for the 21st century

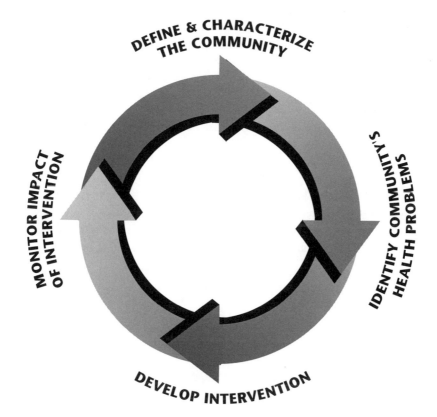

DEFINE & CHARACTERIZE THE COMMUNITY

IDENTIFY COMMUNITY'S HEALTH PROBLEMS

DEVELOP INTERVENTION

MONITOR IMPACT OF INTERVENTION

Edited by
Robert Rhyne, M.D., Richard Bogue, Ph.D.,
Gary Kukulka, Ph.D., Hugh Fulmer, M.D.

American Public Health Association
1015 Fifteenth Street, NW
Washington, DC 20005

American Public Health Association
1015 Fifteenth St., NW
Washington, DC 20005-2605
http://www.apha.org

Mohammad N. Akhter, MD, MPH
Executive Director

2.5M 11/98
Library of Congress Catalog Card Number: 98-74064

ISBN: 0-87553-236-5

Printed and bound in the United States of America.

Cover Design: *Anne Dougherty, A/D Design*

Book Design: *Free Hand Press, Inc. for Magnificent Publications, Inc.*

Typeset in: *Book Antiqua and Futura*

Printing and Binding: *Kirby Lithographic Company, Inc., Arlington, VA*

CONTENTS

Chapter 4: Leadership and Management in COPC 58

Richard Bogue
Richard Roberts
Martin Hickey

Chapter 5: Techniques for Developing a Community Partnership 88

Nina Wallerstein
Barbara Sheline

Chapter 6: Defining and Characterizing Community Denominators

Tom Becker
Robert Rhyne

Chapter 7: Identifying and Characterizing Community Health Problems

Richard Kozoll

Chapter 8: Evaluating Your Intervention

Deborah Helitzer
Robert Rhyne
Betty Skipper
Laurie Kastelic

David Garr
Margaret Kelsey

Chapter 10: Education and Training in Community-Oriented Primary Care 213

Suzanne Cashman
Ron Anderson
Hugh Fulmer

Appendices 238

Index 264

CONTRIBUTORS

Ron I. Anderson, MD
CEO, Parkland Health &
Hospital System
Dallas, Tex

Tom Becker, MD, MPH
Professor
Public Health and
Preventive Medicine
Oregon Health Sciences
University
Portland, Ore

Richard Bogue, PhD
Senior Director of
Governance Programs
American Hospital
Association
Chicago, Ill

Suzanne B. Cashman, DSc
Associate Director
Center for Community
Responsive Care, Inc.
Boston, Mass
and
Private Consultant in
Public Health

David Cockley, DrPH
Assistant Professor,
Health Sciences
James Madison University
Harrisonburg, Va

Frank H. Crespin, MD, MPH
Medical Director
La Clinica de la Familia
Las Cruces, NM

Robert DeVries
Program Director
W.K. Kellogg Foundation
Battle Creek, Mich

Hugh S. Fulmer, MD, MPH
Executive Director
Center for Community
Responsive Care, Inc.
Boston, Mass

David Garr, MD
Associate Dean for
Primary Care
Department of Family
Medicine
Medical University of
South Carolina
Charleston, SC

Linda Hachfeld, MPH, RD
President and Publisher
Appletree Press
Mankato, Minn

L. Clark Hansbarger, MD
Assoc. Dean for Graduate
Medical Education
Associate Professor,
Pediatrics
University of New Mexico
School of Medicine
Albuquerque, NM

Deborah L. Helitzer, ScD
Director, Office of
Evaluation, Center for
Health Promotion
University of New Mexico
School of Medicine
Albuquerque, NM

Martin Hickey, MD
President and CEO
Lovelace Health Systems
Albuquerque, NM

Martin Kantrowitz, MD
Professor Emeritus
University of New Mexico
School of Medicine
Albuquerque, NM

Laurie Kastelic
Program Coordinator
Department of Family and
Community Medicine
University of New Mexico
School of Medicine
Albuquerque, NM

Margaret Heinzerling Kelsey, MPH
Research Assistant
Office of the Associate
Dean for Primary Care
Medical University of
South Carolina
Charleston, SC

Jenny Koinis, RN, MSN
Diabetes Educator
Kaiser Permanente
Durham, NC

Tom Koinis, MD
Private Practice of
Medicine
Stovall Medical Center
Stovall, NC

Richard Kozoll, MD
Private Practitioner
Los Pinos Family Health
Cuba, NM
and
Clinical Professor
Department of Family and
Community Medicine
University of New Mexico
School of Medicine
Albuquerque, NM

Gary Kukulka, PhD
Education and Research
Associate
Department of Family
Practice
Lehigh Valley Hospital
Allentown, Penn

Bill Manahan, MD
Assistant Professor
Department of Family
Medicine
University of Minnesota
School of Medicine
Minneapolis, Minn

Marma McIntee, MS
Family Living Educator
University of
Wisconsin Extension
Washington County
Extension Office
West Bend, Wis

Robert L. Rhyne, MD
Associate Professor
Department of Family and
Community Medicine
University of New Mexico
School of Medicine
Albuquerque, NM

Richard Roberts, MD, JD
Professor
Department of Family
Medicine
University of Wisconsin-
Madison
Madison, Wis

Barbara Sheline, MD, MPH
Assistant Dean for
Primary Care
Duke University Medical
Center
Durham, NC

Betty Skipper, PhD
Professor
Department of Family and
Community Medicine
University of New Mexico
School of Medicine
Albuquerque, NM

Henry G. Taylor, MD
Commissioner
State of West Virginia
Bureau for Public Health
Charleston, WVa

Ben Thompson, MD
Private Practice of
Medicine
Chittenden, Vt

Nina Wallerstein, DrPH
Associate Professor
Director, Masters in Public
Health Program
Department of Family and
Community Medicine
University of New Mexico
School of Medicine
Albuquerque, NM

William H. Wiese, MD, MPH
Director, Public Health
Division
New Mexico Department
of Health
Santa Fe, NM

FOREWORD

The United States' experience with Community-Oriented Primary Care (COPC), while largely limited to the last 40 years, has been dynamic and instructive. This book provides a broad view of the experiences and processes which teams of health professionals and community leaders have faced in addressing a series of health problems for their defined populations. From these experiences has emerged a clear sense of the need for practical skills training in COPC. This book presents instruction in the most critical skills needed by the successful COPC practitioner, illustrated by "real-life" examples of COPC processes, both rural and urban.

Health care at the end of this century is marked by corporate and government demands for improvements expressed particularly through managed care; consolidation of institutional providers into new care systems; broad acceptance of new clinicians such as nurse practitioners; increases in the numbers of uninsured; and threats to the survival of "last resort" health providers such as public hospitals, neighborhood health centers, and inner city-serving academic health centers. With the continued need to guard and ensure the public's health regardless of the changes taking place, this publication is timely, since COPC techniques continue to prove their worth in this rapidly changing environment.

This book shows how to employ COPC methods and skills for cost effective, accessible, high quality health care for a recognized population. The authors emphasize:

1. The concentration of methods and interventions on population-derived health needs (rather than institutional problems and agendas), with particular attention to care of the underserved;

2. COPC insistence on the full engagement of a host of community leaders (such as schools, agencies on aging, business coalitions for health), with key health professionals involved in identifying the problems and solutions;

3. Health promotion and disease prevention as part of the overall reorganization of health services;

4. Primary care over tertiary, acute, inpatient hospital care;

5. Greater involvement of the public health sector;

6. Problem solving and reorganization, both community-wide and multi-professional; and

7. Understanding how COPC values can complement managed care and community benefit programs for the 21st century.

Today's clinical training and practice are changing rapidly. The consolidation of services into comprehensive care systems lends itself well to COPC values. Students in the health professions now learn they have two "patients"—the individual and the community. Community benefit programs that are now required in seven states insist on new relationships between health providers and community leadership—relationships beyond the diagnosis and treatment of the individual patient. Managed care plans are bound to see the value of COPC. Will the licensing and accreditation of these managed care plans soon suggest a problem solving approach such as COPC?

Public health practice in America continues to be challenged, restructured, and redefined. This book offers new, realistic insight into how medicine, health systems, non-health community leaders, and social services can be supportive of these changes. Solid COPC approaches ensure that priority health needs are addressed in a timely manner with "buy-in" by all key segments of the community.

—*Robert A. DeVries, Program Director*
W.K. Kellogg Foundation, Battle Creek, Mich

PREFACE

This book grew out of the authors' experiences with the Community Oriented Primary Care (COPC) process in many sites throughout the US and their belief that utilizing practical skills is as important to success as is theory. Not having had an "instruction manual" on how to approach COPC challenged the authors continually to try, readjust, retool, rethink, and reassess when approaching the practicalities of COPC. They learned valuable lessons and gained insight into the Institute of Medicine (IOM) model of COPC. By sharing what they know with those new to COPC, the authors hope to improve the newcomers' chances of success.

Many of the authors' experiences in this book were gained through their participation in the Community-Oriented Primary Care National Rural Demonstration Project (1988-1991) and the Urban COPC Demonstration Project (1988-1993). Both of these groundbreaking projects were funded by the W.K. Kellogg Foundation of Battle Creek, Mich. In addition, many authors have a depth of additional COPC experience, either as health care providers or administrators.

The National Rural Demonstration Project was administered jointly by the National Rural Health Association and the Hospital Research and Educational Trust of the American Hospital Association. Thirteen rural sites representing a broad spectrum of health care facilities and professional programs were selected to participate in the project, which required adherence to the classical four steps of COPC, as well as community involvement (see Appendix 1.1).

Each site received funding for a three-year cycle of designing, implementing, and evaluating a COPC process. Each had access to professional technical assistance through a consulting arrangement with the University of New Mexico School of Medicine, which held an initial training session and a culminating debriefing session for all sites, in addition to assigning one-on-one consultants to each site for the duration of the project. Many "snapshots" of the sites' experiences are provided as chapter examples.

The urban COPC demonstration, entitled the "Community Health Initiative," was administered by the Carney Hospital in Boston, a teaching hospital allied with a network of community health centers serving the urban neighborhoods of Dorchester, Mattapan, and South Boston. The Codman Square and Bowdoin Street health centers were selected as sites for special emphasis.

At these sites, community organizing and involvement became essential ingredients in the development of a community-based, problem-focused health services system. In contrast to the rural demonstration, the urban initiative flowed from structuring a training model, based at the hospital and health center network, that included faculty development (with a grant from the Health Resources and Services Administration) and preventive medicine residency/fellowship (supported by Medicare graduate medical education funding) in COPC. This way, the concept of community involvement in COPC was built in from the onset. The demonstration featured health professionals already skilled as clinicians learning how to involve communities as partners and becoming, together, capable of caring for whole communities.

Of the many lessons that emerged from the authors' experiences with COPC, a few stood out above the rest:

▶ The COPC process takes longer than expected.

▶ Funding helps build and sustain projects.

▶ A primary care practice does not need to be the pivotal element of COPC.

▶ COPC can be practiced in a variety of settings both urban and rural.

▶ Evaluation is difficult because few have training in how to approach the process.

▶ Training in COPC should become a standard.

▶ COPC can be both rewarding and stressful.

The authors have also learned how integral sustained community involvement is to the COPC process, and that a dedicated, well-trained corps of community people can be invaluable in developing and sustaining a successful COPC project. Of all the lessons learned, perhaps this is the strongest: building a strong sense of community esteem and competence in addressing its identified problems is the enduring legacy of COPC. In fact, the model of COPC in this book includes five, not four, steps of COPC; the additional step is "involve the community." The other four steps of the classic IOM model are retained: defining and characterizing the community, selecting a health problem to address in the community, designing an intervention to change some aspect of the problem and improve the health of the community, and evaluating the intervention and monitoring the process.

The authors' experience of being allowed to observe people's firsthand COPC experiences during the Kellogg-funded COPC projects and others' experiences with COPC sites was very rewarding, and it led to the decision that a manual of practical COPC skills was sorely needed. The seed for this book was planted. It would take the reflections of many people, including four editors with strong COPC backgrounds and experiences, numerous authors who participated in the demonstration projects as either consultants or site project directors, and site representatives who contributed vignettes, to synthesize and distill the experiences into practical skills. Participants in Kellogg demonstration projects and other COPC project sites across the country gave life to this book; we thank them for welcoming us into their communities and for their willingness to share their experiences, both good and bad, that helped in the formation of the skills presented in this book.

In writing this book, the authors sought to provide a complete set of COPC skills for the health professional who needs to be able to access these skills quickly and learn the basics of COPC in a brief amount of reading time. Topics are presented in a stepwise fashion, which allows the reader to review discrete chapters as needed without relying heavily on material from other chapters. (Of course, we suggest that the entire book be read—there are valuable lessons in every chapter!) Topics include determining whether or not to do COPC (Chapter 2), building a COPC team (Chapter 3), performing the skills central to the five steps of COPC (Chapters 5-8), and sustaining successful efforts (Chapter 9). A chapter outlining basic leadership and management skills has been included (Chapter 4) because most health professionals are not trained in these skills, and the lack of these skills can lead to the downfall of a COPC process. Finally, a chapter addressing techniques for incorporating COPC education into the training of health care professionals is included (Chapter 10).

R.R.
R.B.
G.K.
H.F.

ACKNOWLEDGMENTS

Special thanks go to the American Public Health Association Publications Division, especially Dorothy Oda, the APHA liaison for this work; Berttina Wentworth, Chair of the APHA Publications Board during the development of this book; Ellen Meyer, Director of Publications, APHA; and Sabine Beisler, former Director of Publications, APHA. Their belief in the need for this book, and their patience in waiting while the editors compiled a book they could be proud of, merit the authors' most sincere thanks.

Also, the editors would like to thank Suzanne Cashman, DSc, Associate Director of the Center for Community-Responsive Care, Inc. in Boston, for her astute contributions as manuscript reviewer and author of numerous chapter examples. Her work was thorough and insightful, and she could be counted on for prompt attention to any task she undertook, with professional and thoughtful results.

We also thank our authors who have made the commitment to COPC for "the long haul." They endured many drafts, reviewers' comments, and editorial changes in the writings. Without their efforts, there would have been no book.

Other associates have helped perform much of the research and coordination involved in compiling the book. Special thanks go to Laurie Kastelic, who coordinated communications among APHA, editors, and authors. She reviewed multiple manuscripts and gave constructive criticism. Her contributions in organization, editing, typing, proofreading, research, and trouble-shooting made this process run smoothly. We would also like to thank Cheri Koinis for her research into the history of COPC and assisting with coordination of UNM consultant team efforts during the rural demonstration project.

To others who may not have been mentioned but who contributed in "behind-the-scenes" fashion, we thank you, also. We hope you will see your contributions reflected in the pages of this book.

CHAPTER 1

An Introduction to Community-Oriented Primary Care (COPC)

Robert Rhyne

Suzanne Cashman

Martin Kantrowitz

ABSTRACT

Community-Oriented Primary Care (COPC) is a systematic process for identifying and addressing the health problems of a defined population. It can be implemented with the resources available in most communities. In COPC, a team of health professionals and community members work in partnership over a long period, diagnosing and treating a community in much the same way as does a primary care physician with an individual patient. Primary care practitioners are not required in every project, and they are usually too busy to lead such an effort, but they must be involved. The roots of COPC date back to the mid-19th century. The authors present a five-step model of the process: (1) define and characterize the community, (2) involve the community, (3) identify community health problems, (4) develop an intervention, and (5) monitor the impact of the intervention. The feedback loop for obtaining results of an intervention is typically short. Because it measures outcomes, COPC will continue to grow in importance in a managed care environment. By engaging in COPC, a health professional can gain not only personal satisfaction but the knowledge needed to reduce future occurrences of specific illnesses and to become a superior performer under managed care. This book, which draws extensively on the authors' personal experiences, is a compendium of skills covering all aspects of the COPC process.

COPC AND THE DAWN OF MANAGED CARE

As a new millennium approaches, health professionals are being asked to change their ways of caring for people. Managed care emphasizes and scrutinizes outcomes of care as never before. This change was stimulated by spiraling health care costs dating back to the end of World War II and by a belief that the crisis might be solved through a business management approach.

A related development is our growing awareness, through instantaneous worldwide communications, of health problems that occur in populations, such as the HIV epidemic, violence and domestic abuse, unwanted pregnancy among teens, and drug abuse. In its report *Healthy People 2000* the US Public Health Service has established national goals for addressing some of these problems.[1]

During this time of tumultuous change, we have an opportunity to expand our vision of health care to include both primary care and population health. With this new vision, we can help to meet national objectives while improving the health of our communities. Some have proposed COPC as a method of integrating managed care, primary care, and population health.[2] We endorse this view. We regard COPC as a logical, common-sense process that can be implemented with tools and personnel available in most communities.

WHAT IS COPC?

COPC is a process by which a defined population's health problems are systematically identified and addressed.[3,4] Ideally, it combines principles of primary care, epidemiology, and public health. There is nothing special about the name; the process could be called community-responsive health care, community-based primary care, or something else. The process is the important element. The community is a partner at every step.

In COPC, a team of community representatives and health professionals is assembled. Its composition can be fluid, with people participating as time and interest allow, as long as a core membership takes responsibility for developing and maintaining the process. The team selects a health problem and designs an intervention and evaluation plan. If its efforts are successful, the team can go on to address other problems. The process can extend over years and can address a host of community problems.

Just as a health care provider uses a specific clinical process to care for an individual, the COPC team uses a specific process to identify and treat community problems. As shown in Table 1.1, both involve similar steps.[4]

COPC focuses on a defined population within a community, making its scope broader than that of a traditional medical practice, which concentrates on the care of individual patients, but narrower than the scope of most epidemiologic studies. A COPC process could focus on:

▶ Geographically defined populations such as a town or county;

▶ Specific population groups, such as infants and their mothers, school-age children, or the elderly; or

▶ People congregated at particular sites, such as the workplace.[5,6]

The community perspective in COPC is a new focus for most health professionals. Considering populations such as those above as "patients" in need of medical services—entities in which specific health problems can be identified and addressed—presents an exciting challenge. Most medical knowledge about population risk factors and disease comes from large epidemiological studies reported in medical or public health journals and the news media. These studies often take five to 10 years from inception to reporting. In contrast to this long feedback loop, the time it takes a COPC team to implement an intervention and report back to the community can often be measured in months rather than years (see Figure 1.1).[7] With feedback so immediate, the COPC team can modify the intervention if no beneficial change is found, or it can institutionalize a successful intervention and monitoring plan.

COPC's systematic approach helps one think logically through all the steps of a project before beginning. COPC requires long range planning and development of methods for data collection, analysis, and reporting of results to the community and the COPC team. It requires that the team plan ahead and anticipate obstacles to successful completion of the project. The key to managing the long-term process is repeated population-based measurement.

TABLE 1.1
Complementary Functions of Clinical Care and Community-Oriented Primary Care

CLINICAL: Individual	COPC: Population
Examination of a patient Interview and examination of individuals using history, physical examination, and laboratory, x-ray and other testing techniques.	**Community Survey** State of health of community and families, using local opinion, secondary data sources, questionnaires, physical, psychological and laboratory testing.
Diagnosis 1. Usually of a patient complaint using differential diagnoses to determine main cause of patient's complaint. 2. Appraisal of health status of a "well" person, such as a pregnant woman, well children, periodic health examinations of adults.	**Community Diagnosis** 1. Usually problem-oriented. Higher frequency of a particular condition in the community and its causes. 2. Health status of the community as a whole or of defined segments of it, e.g., health of expectant mothers, growth and development of children, birth and death rates.
Treatment 1. According to diagnosis and depending on resources of patient and medical institutions. 2. Intervention usually follows for the patient seeking care for illness or advice about health.	**Treatment** 1. According to the community diagnosis and depending on resources of health services system and community. 2. Population intervention to prevent/treat specific diseases or reduce risk.
Monitoring Therapy 1. Evaluation of patient's progress and response to treatment. 2. Ongoing treatment of chronic illnesses, e.g., hypertension.	**Evaluation** 1. Evaluation of intervention programs and COPC process. Surveillance of health indicators in community. 2. Incorporation of community treatment into community health care system.

Adapted from Kark SL. *The Practice of Community-Oriented Primary Health Care.* New York: Appleton-Century-Crofts; 1981.

WHY DO COPC?

There are many reasons to become involved in COPC. Most health professionals have been trained to focus only on individual patients, and COPC broadens their perspective. Many find it intellectually stimulating to learn new skills for managing a population's health. It is rewarding to become involved in one's community and gain new perspective on what happens there. Most health care professionals feel an altruistic "calling" that can be extended to their community. COPC can fulfill this need by reducing suffering throughout an entire community. COPC can also prepare practitioners for superior performance in a managed care environment, in which they may be asked to monitor parameters in their practices. If you are already used to collecting data and evaluating outcome indicators via COPC, this will not be a foreign concept.

COPC's greatest potential may lie in its capacity to help health professionals influence the future. Health care resources are becoming more constrained. The baby boomers will soon reach their chronic disease years. The nation's payment systems continue shifting toward capitation and other mechanisms for focusing financial risk. The ideology and practice of COPC represent core knowledge for tomorrow's health care practitioner. In particular, the knowledge needed to reduce future occurrences of specific illnesses will be in great demand. The practitioners who design tomorrow's community health systems will be those who learn how to:

- ▶ Measure health problems relative to a specific population;

- ▶ Work collaboratively to identify, characterize, and prioritize a community's health problems;

- ▶ Solicit low-cost or voluntary community assistance in designing, creating, and implementing interventions; and

- ▶ Quantify and communicate future savings, in terms of better health outcomes and lower costs.

HISTORY OF COPC: FROM CHOLERA PREVENTION TO WORLDWIDE INITIATIVE

As we discuss the COPC process, it is important to distinguish between COPC and primary care. Primary care, as the Institute of Medicine (IOM) of the National Academy of Sciences defined it in 1978 and in a 1994 revision,

FIGURE 1.1: Long and Short Information Feedback Loops

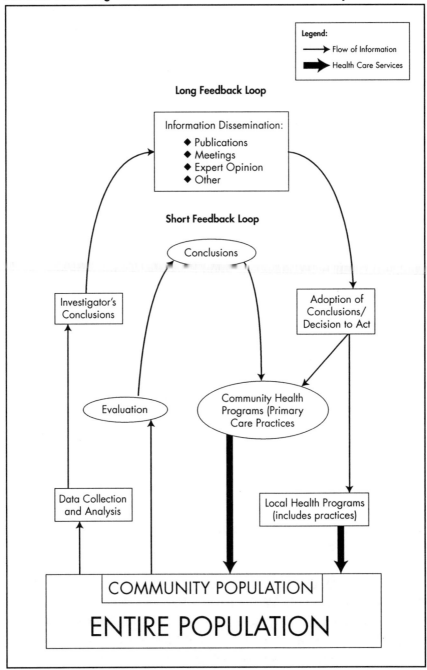

Adapted from Mullan F and Nutting PA, Primary care epidemiology: new users of old tools. *Family Medicine.* 1986;18:221-225.

is that form of care that is continuous, accessible, comprehensive, coordinated, and accountable.[8] The World Health Organization (WHO) conference in Alma Ata, USSR, defined primary care in 1978 as "care that includes the provision of promotive, preventive, curative, and rehabilitative services and, specifically, education regarding health problems, promotion of proper nutrition, safe water, and basic sanitation."[9] The WHO definition is much broader and encompasses the needs of developing countries. While the WHO definition may seem to fit better with ideal COPC principles, most American health care providers think of primary care in terms of the IOM definition, and that is the definition we follow in this book. The 1994 IOM definition incorporates aspects of COPC by stating that primary care practitioners should practice in the context of family and community.[10]

At present in the US, COPC is not primary care in either the IOM or WHO sense. It has evolved into something quite different, an approach focused specifically on a defined community. Nutting, in his early writing, stated that a primary care practice was a necessary ingredient in COPC.[9] At that time, the intent was to join primary care with public health and epidemiology. Indeed, COPC is not meant to be primary care for a community. The "PC" is included because COPC's founders envisioned it originating and being led by primary care practitioners.[11] Experience has shown that COPC can be practiced in a variety of other settings as well, including hospitals and public health departments, health centers, and academic centers. COPC is actually a means to empower a community to address selected problems using a logical, systematic approach.

Historically, community participation has been part of many efforts to improve health. John Snow, a British medical doctor, became the first to apply a team approach and epidemiologic techniques when, in 1855, he discovered that a local water company was the source of a cholera epidemic in London.[12] Since the late 1880s, community organizers and social workers have promoted community participation in health issues in the context of improved housing and services, better jobs, healthier workplaces, and safer neighborhoods.[13]

Community-Oriented Primary Care as it is currently conceived was practiced as early as the 1930s, when community physicians incorporated elements of epidemiology into their practices.[14,15] Dr. Will Pickles systematically recorded the name, date, residence, and diagnosis of patients who presented to his practice during an infectious disease epidemic. For assistance, he enlisted a "community care team" that included his family, patients, the Minister of Health, epidemiologists, a geologist, a photographer, schoolteachers, and the clergy. The accomplishments of Will Pickles were really those of a primary care physician leading a team of concerned community members and health professionals to solve a community health problem.

The notion of COPC was first codified in the 1940s by Dr. Sidney Kark. He and his wife, Dr. Emily Kark, originated the concept of "Community-Oriented Primary Health Care" (COPHC) while practicing in Pholela, South Africa, with a Zulu tribe.[4,5] After diagnosing nutritional problems such as kwashiorkor and pellagra, they established community health centers, surveyed patients' dietary habits, and provided nutrition education. The resulting changes in eating habits led to a reduction in kwashiorkor.[16] The current definition of COPC was derived from the Karks' experience with COPHC, in which they extended the practice of primary care from purely clinical to epidemiologic and community aspects of care.[1]

The first COPC initiative in the United States began in the 1950s, when the US Public Health Service contracted with Cornell Medical School's Department of Public Health for a comprehensive program of primary care and community health services for Native Americans.[17] The initiative led to the Navajo-Cornell Field Health Research Project in Many Farms, Arizona, whose staff of physicians, nurses, social scientists, and Navajos worked as a team to respond to community needs. Community involvement was a *sine qua non* of the project, which provided opportunities for researchers, clinicians, and medical students to develop an appreciation for COPC. The Navajo-Cornell project director, Kurt Deuschle, went on to establish the first Department of Community Medicine in 1960. It was based at the University of Kentucky and patterned after the Navajo-Cornell project.[18-21]

By the 1960s, community participation was required for federally funded community health centers in the US, a mandate which continues to this day.[22] Community-wide cardiovascular interventions in Northern California, Rhode Island, Minnesota, and North Karelia, Finland, successfully used community participation to improve health outcomes.[23,24] And the Centers for Disease Control implemented its first Planned Approach to Community Health (PATCH) program in 1984, involving community-wide data collection and decision-making throughout the United States (but not necessarily involving local health professionals).[25,26] Subsequently, the following federal efforts incorporated the COPC approach: Healthy Communities 2000[1], Assessment Protocol for Excellence in Public Health (APEX)[27], and the National Civic League's Healthy Cities.[28]

At the Alma Ata conference in 1978, the WHO renewed a call to make community participation an essential element in individual and community health, with power and responsibility shared equally between community members and health professionals.[9] At the first international conference on health promotion in 1986, the Ottawa Charter expanded the view of health promotion to a participatory process in which individuals and communities increase their control over the determinants of health. Since 1986 the WHO Healthy Cities Project has attracted over 400 cities worldwide to implement policies of community participation, health equity, and multisectoral agency collaboration to create healthier environments.[29]

In 1982, the IOM sponsored a conference on Community-Oriented Primary Care with participants from many different sites around the United States and six foreign countries.[30] They all shared an interest in health care programs that tailored a primary care practice or health program to the health needs of a defined population; most had experience implementing COPC in some form. From this conference, a study group was formed to develop an operational model for the US. Their work, published in 1984, provided an operational definition of COPC and reported on seven case studies that provided empirical data on its everyday practice.[8]

The IOM report represents a benchmark in the development of COPC.[8,30] For the first time in the US, a distinguished group of scholars and practitioners studied the concept of COPC, examined what was known about its operations, costs, and impacts, and made recommendations about future work on this practice modality. Based on the literature as well as the 1982 conference's work, the committee developed an operational definition of COPC and used it as a basis for organizing site visits. Study sites had to meet the following criteria: 1) they had to have an active medical practice emphasizing primary care; 2) the practice had to assume responsibility for the health care of a defined community—beyond active users of the practice; and 3) there had to be systematic efforts to identify the community and address its major health problems. Through observations at seven sites, the committee concluded that, while COPC was not the prevailing mode of practice, the conceptual model held promise. They urged that COPC be implemented in a variety of clinical settings so that its impact on health status and costs could be studied.

Since the IOM study, others have examined the skills necessary to practice COPC.[3,31-34] The University of California School of Public Health at Berkeley, through a grant from the Bureau of Health Care Delivery and Assistance, in 1988 published a COPC practice manual for primary care settings, based on their experience with field projects in San Francisco.[31] The American Academy of Family Physicians published a monograph entitled Community-Oriented Primary Care as part of its Home Study Self-Assessment course.[32] The US Department of Health and Human Services (DHHS) published a compilation of strategies in *Community-Oriented Primary Care: From Principle to Practice*,[3] edited by Nutting.

In 1987 the W.K. Kellogg Foundation funded the National Rural Health Association (NRHA) and the Hospital Research and Educational Trust (HRET) to perform a demonstration project in which 13 rural sites would develop the practice of COPC (Appendix 1.1). A year later, the Foundation funded an urban COPC demonstration program. While the publications cited above contain certain skills necessary for the COPC process, none could provide the practitioners in these demonstration projects with a complete, accessible compendium of skills that covered all aspects of the COPC process. This book attempts to meet that need.

A NEW OPERATIONAL MODEL

In a two-volume report entitled *COPC: A Practical Assessment*,[8,30] published in 1984 by the Institute of Medicine, Nutting *et al* presented a four-step operational model. The report included staging criteria for determining whether each step was being carried out in practice and concluded that no fully operational models of COPC were being practiced in any of the study sites. The authors encouraged the development and testing of methods to perform COPC and move existing primary care practices toward COPC.

After many years of practical experience, the authors of this book now propose changes in the model that will bring it into line with COPC at its best. Most important, we think it is critical to articulate five steps instead of four. While the definition developed by Nutting *et al* listed four steps, the narrative defined COPC as a "process by which the practice, *with the participation of the community,* identifies and addresses the major health problems of the community" (italics added).[8] Indeed, a minority opinion in the report suggested that community involvement be included as "one of the key structural components of COPC." We also view community participation as key; with it, we move from doing "to and for" to functioning "in, with, and by" a community. When professionals work with community members from the start, community ownership will be established.

Thus, we propose a new, five-stage model—with staging criteria for the new second step—that otherwise follows the Nutting criteria (Table 1.2):

TABLE 1.2
Five-Step Operational Model for COPC
with Staging Criteria for Community Involvement Step

Step 1:   Define and Characterize the Community

Step 2:   Involve the Community

Stage 0: No effort is made to organize or involve the community in the site's work or to get community input.

Stage I: The importance of community involvement is recognized but efforts of outreach to the community are limited and their participation is superficial.

Stage II: Systematic efforts are made to invite the community to participate in and be oriented to the COPC process. Although broad-based community input is encouraged, only a few well-recognized community leaders are involved.

Stage III: The community is organized and participates in the process but is not perceived as an equal partner by either the professionals or itself.

Stage IV: Extensive and formal ongoing outreach takes place. Community members, recognized leaders as well as grassroots citizens, participate in all aspects of the COPC process. The community members and the professionals view each other as valued partners.

Step 3:   Identify Community Health Problems

Step 4:   Develop Intervention

Step 5:   Monitor Impact of Intervention

Experience has shown that the steps are not mutually exclusive and often cannot be performed in consecutive order. The order may vary depending on the community, the exact health problem, and the approach taken by the COPC team. In practice, one needs to move back and forth among the major steps, as shown in Figure 1.2.

FIGURE 1.2: The COPC Process

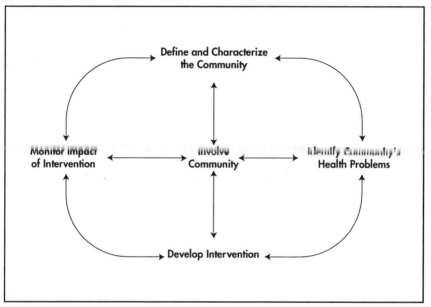

THE COPC PROCESS

To illustrate: Let's say you compile a thorough set of demographic and socioeconomic data using the most recent census and use this information to characterize the community, initiate community involvement, and rally local support for the COPC process. Then you move on to identifying the first community problem on which to work. Say your team decides on cardiovascular risk reduction in the workplace. Instead of designing an intervention (the next step in the model), logic suggests that you next characterize the chosen workplace community denominator, which requires revisiting the community definition and characterization step. In the dynamic process of COPC, you may revisit earlier steps to refine and readjust your plan many times as you focus in on a particular community, involve community members in the process, decide on an aspect of a problem to address, design an intervention, and devise an evaluation system.

We therefore propose two further modifications to the original model articulated by Nutting and the Institute of Medicine. Besides adding the step "Involve the community," we propose that the steps be seen not as sequential but as dynamic and capable of being revisited as needed as the team goes through the COPC process.

The third proposed modification involves the relationship of COPC to primary care practices. Nutting suggested that, in order for COPC to be practiced, three components had to be present: a primary care practice, a defined community population, and a process for designing and implementing health intervention in a community.[13,33] We have found that COPC can be practiced successfully in settings other than primary care practices, for example, managed care organizations, hospitals, public health departments, and other agencies. However, it is necessary to involve a primary care practice in the overall COPC process, just not in each individual project. Health professionals in the COPC process can help the team understand medical problems and bring credibility to the process. We, therefore, believe that Nutting's first component should be changed to "involve community members and health professionals."

In order to improve the health status of a community, medical practices must become more responsive to the community's needs. Clinical expertise is essential, but the administrators of COPC need not be clinically focused. In fact, the administration of COPC often works better if the day-to-day decision making and operations are not performed by physicians, who are usually too busy to coordinate COPC efforts. If resources permit, it is best to have a dedicated COPC coordinator administer the process and coordinate the efforts of the team. Chapters 2 and 3 will expand on the role of the health professional in the COPC process.

The model of COPC continues to evolve. The model initiated by Kark and modified by Nutting provided an essential starting place. Experience with it has led us to suggest the modifications discussed, and other suggestions for changing our concepts of COPC are likely to be made as experience builds.

THIS BOOK: A COMPENDIUM FOR PRACTITIONERS

This book represents a complete, accessible compendium of skills covering all aspects of the COPC process. Its contents are drawn from previous publications as well as the authors' personal experiences observing many different sites where COPC has been practiced. As a reference work, the book can be consulted one chapter at a time as needed. Not all skills will be required at every site; they can be adapted to each community's needs.

As stated earlier, we consider COPC a logical, common-sense effort and a smart business move that can be accomplished in most communities. We believe that time and effort are well spent on COPC regardless of how elaborate the effort or how far the process goes. While the ultimate goal of COPC is to demonstrate that health interventions have an impact, COPC has other advantages. It can also build a sense of community. It enables the COPC team to do the most good at the least cost, and it encourages empowerment of community and health sectors alike in solving community-wide health problems. For some practitioners, COPC may be only a modification or extension of current practice; for others, it will be a real change.

REFERENCES

1. US Department of Health and Human Services, Public Health Service. *Healthy People 2000: National Health Promotion and Disease Prevention Objectives: Summary.* Sudbury, MA: Jones and Bartlett Publishers; 1992.
2. Wright R. Community oriented primary care: the cornerstone of health care reform. *JAMA.* 1993;269:2544-2547.
3. Nutting PA. *Community-Oriented Primary Care: From Principle to Practice.* Washington, DC: US Department of Health and Human Services, Health Resources and Services Administration; 1987; 86-1:xv.
4. Kark SL. *The Practice of Community-Oriented Primary Health Care.* New York, NY: Appleton-Century-Crofts; 1981.
5. Kark SL, Kark E. An alternative strategy in community-oriented primary health care. *Israel J Med Sciences.* 1980;19:707-713.
6. Abramson JH, Kark SL. Community-focused health care: introduction. *Israel J Med Sciences.* 1981;17:65-70.
7. Mullan F. Community-oriented primary care: epidemiology's role in the future of primary care. *Public Health Reports.* 1984;99:442-443.
8. Nutting PA, Connor EM, eds. Institute of Medicine. *Community-Oriented Primary Care: A Practical Assessment.* Washington, DC: National Academy Press; 1984;1.
9. Health for All Series. *Primary Health Care: Report of the International Conference on Primary Health Care, Alma Ata.* Geneva, Switzerland: World Health Organization; 1978;1.
10. Donaldson MS, et al, eds. *Primary Care: America's Health in a New Era.* Washington, DC: National Academy Press; 1996.
11. Nutting PA, Conner P. Community-oriented primary care: an examination of the US experience. *AJPH.* 1986;76:279-281.

12. Mausner JA, Bahn AK. *Epidemiology: An Introductory Text*. Philadelphia, Penn: WB Sanders; 1974.
13. Minkler M. Improving health through community organization. In: Glanz K, Lewis FM, Rimer B, eds. *Health Behavior and Health Education: Theory, Research and Practice*. San Francisco, Calif: Jossey-Bass Publishers; 1990.
14. Pickles WN. *Epidemiology in Country Practice*. Bristol, England: John Wright and Sons, Ltd; 1939;23-29.
15. Mettee TM. William N. Pickles, MD: a country doctor with a naturalist's interest in illness. In: Nutting PA, ed. *Community-Oriented Primary Care: From Principle to Practice*. Washington, DC: US Department of Health and Human Services, Health Resources and Services Administration; 1987; 86-1: chap. 1.
16. Kark SL, Steuart GW, eds. *A Practice of Social Medicine*. Edinburgh, Scotland: E & S Livingstone Ltd; 1962.
17. McDermott W, Deuschle K, Adair J, Fulmer H, Loughlin B. Introducing modern medicine in a Navajo community. *Science*. 1960;131:197-205, 280-289.
18. Deuschle K, Fulmer H. Community medicine: a new department at the University of Kentucky. *J Med Educ*. 1962;37:434-45.
19. Deuschle K, Fulmer H, McNamara M, Tapp J. The Kentucky experiment in community medicine. *Milbank Memorial Fund Quarterly*. 1966;XLIV:9-21.
20. Deuschle K. Community oriented primary care: lessons learned in three decades. *J Community Hlth*. 1982;8:13-22.
21. Fulmer H. Teaching community medicine in Kentucky. *Harvard School of Public Health Alumni Bulletin*. 1994;21:2-6.
22. Geiger J. Community health centers: health care as an instrument of social change. In: Sidel V, Sidel R, eds. *Reforming Medicine: Lessons of the Last Quarter Century*. New York, NY: Pantheon; 1984.
23. Leittaanmaki L, Koskela K, Puska P, McAlister A. The role of lay workers in community health education: experiences of the North Karelia project. *Scandinavian J Social Med*. 1980;8:1-7.
24. Matarazzo J, Miller N, Weiss S, Herd J, eds. *Behavioral Health: A Handbook of Health Enhancement and Disease Prevention*. Silver Spring, Md: John Wiley & Sons; 1984.
25. Nelson CF, et al. Planned approach to community health: the PATCH program. In: Nutting PA, ed. *Community Oriented Primary Care: From Principle to Practice*. Washington, DC: US Department of Health and Human Services, Health Resources and Services Administration; 1987; 86-1: chap. 47.
26. Fulmer H, Cashman S, Hattis P, Schlaff A, Horgan D. Bridging the gap between medicine, public health and the community: PATCH and the Carney Hospital experience. *J Med Educ*. 1992;23:167-70.
27. National Association of County Health Officials. 1991 APEX/PH. *Assessment Protocol for Excellence in Public Health*. Washington, DC: NACHO.
28. Norris T, Lampe D. Healthy communities, healthy people: a challenge of coordination and compassion. *National Civic Review*. 1994;83:280-89.
29. Tsouros AD, ed. *World Health Organization Healthy Cities Project: A Project Becomes a Movement. Review of Progress 1987 to 1990*. Copenhagen, Denmark: Fadl Publishers; 1991.
30. Nutting PA, Connor EM, eds. Institute of Medicine. *Community-Oriented Primary Care: A Practical Assessment*. Washington, DC: National Academy Press; 1984;2.
31. Overall NA, Williamson J, eds. *Community-Oriented Primary Care in Action: A Practice Manual for Primary Care Settings*. University of California at Berkeley School of Public Health; 1988.
32. Nutting PA, Garr DR. Community Oriented Primary Care. Kansas City, Mo: American Academy of Family Physicians; 1989; *Home Study Self-Assessment Working Paper 124*.
33. Nutting PA. Community-oriented primary care: a promising innovation in primary care. *Public Health Reports*. 1985;100:1:3-4.
34. Boufford JI, Shonubi PA. Community-Oriented Primary Care: Training for Urban Practice. New York, NY: *Praeger Special Studies*; 1986.

CHAPTER 2

To Do or Not to Do COPC: Tailoring COPC to Your Setting

William Wiese

Clark Hansbarger

ABSTRACT

A health professional can assess his or her ability to engage in COPC using a number of factors, which will point towards a level of involvement ranging from minimal to large-scale. Prerequisites for an individual and his or her organization include: community-oriented perspectives and values, commitment to long-range (strategic) planning, community involvement, willingness to quantify problems and outcomes, adequate resources, and the likelihood of a positive economic impact. Other conditions also favor success. The COPC process should be seen as relevant by the health organization as well as by the community. The process should be clearly feasible and affordable. The health organization should be financially stable and effectively governed, and it should be delivering adequate quality of care. Staff should feel satisfied and rewarded for their contributions to COPC. Health professionals' peer groups should also value the goals of the COPC effort. Equally important, the COPC team should structure projects to fit within available resources and build upon the health organization's current objectives. Success breeds success, so starting with small efforts and early successes can lead to larger ones.

INTRODUCTION

The practice of COPC can be rewarding and enlightening. It opens new avenues into one's community and provides a new appreciation for health problems on a community scale. However, most people in positions to contemplate becoming involved in a COPC process are already engaged in other activities, for example, as managers of a health care organization or clinicians in busy practices. Undertaking a COPC process will mean adjusting goals, embarking on new activities, forming new relationships and partnerships, and placing demands on scarce resources. In its full expression, the methodology of COPC requires an intensity of focus that may seem incompatible to many who face other demands. Indeed, COPC is not for everyone. Most basically, it requires an interest in the health and well-being of the *population* being served. It also requires a deliberate well-planned approach, a willingness to evaluate the outcomes of one's efforts critically, and a willingness to relinquish some control over the process.

Becoming involved in community-based planning and learning the skills of COPC as presented in this book can improve the practice of most health professionals. COPC skills may also be helpful in areas such as interdisciplinary processes, public health, outcomes management, and core business functions.

We want to help you reduce limitations and barriers, to make the process less mysterious, and to encourage you to gain confidence through community-oriented experiences. This chapter provides guidance on when to launch a new COPC initiative or expand an existing community-based initiative into COPC. In this chapter, we emphasize the need to match COPC objectives with available time, resources, and interest. In particular, we examine the prerequisites for COPC, issues of scale, importance of building on what already exists, and conditions that favor success.

PREREQUISITES: ARE YOU AND YOUR ORGANIZATION READY?

Before venturing into COPC, look at Table 2.1 and explore these issues candidly with the other leaders of your organization. These are issues that the organizational leadership should discuss thoroughly before committing to COPC. Indeed, this exploration of one's own values and attitudes *is* the first step in the COPC process.

TABLE 2.1
Checklist of Prerequisites for COPC

1. **Community-oriented perspectives and values.** Do you value the community as a unit of care? Are you willing to see a project through to completion?

2. **Commitment to long-range (strategic) planning.** Can you set goals, identify and prioritize health problems, carry out a plan to address them, and evaluate the results?

3. **Community involvement.** Do you want to learn the skills of community organization? Are you willing to give up control of the process to a COPC team involving community members? Do you want to develop a "partnership" with the community?

4. **Willingness to quantify.** Do you appreciate the value of monitoring a community intervention using objective, quantitative data?

5. **Resources.** Are you willing to devote time from your already busy schedule, energy and money to support a COPC process? Can you work with other agencies and organizations to develop resources?

6. **Economic impact.** Are your plans compatible with the long-term financial viability of your organization? Will they enhance viability?

1.   **Community-oriented perspectives and values.** All participants in COPC, particularly leadership figures such as board members, health professionals, administrators, and involved community leaders, must assign high value to the health of the community. While this may seem obvious, it cannot be taken for granted. The imperative to care for individuals can easily and indefinitely overwhelm COPC activities, especially when people are busy. COPC requires that you look past the proverbial trees (the individual patients) to see the forest (the community).

COPC requires time, effort and will. Organizational leadership must be willing to design objective analyses, collect and analyze data on the outcomes of the services provided, and examine the unmet health needs in the community. Clinicians must be willing to change established patterns of practice.

It is not enough to value a community-oriented approach to health. This must be coupled with a spirit of activism and involvement. Awareness of community health problems must be followed by active steps of analysis, data collection, and interaction with people and agencies, all of which lead to programmatic intervention and evaluation. The spirit of activism provides the energy for building resources and coalitions and bypassing or tearing down old barriers. Successful COPC projects can take considerable time to accomplish and usually require tenacity and perseverance.

A broad base of interest among professional staff and in the community will help in building support and commitment. Those with initial interest must determine the degree of enthusiasm among others. The most direct way is to ask. Meetings, individual discussions, and surveys may be appropriate.

2.   Commitment to long-range (strategic) planning. Don't be turned off by the phrase "strategic planning." It usually causes health professionals to sound the "jargon alert," but it is neither a complicated nor a difficult idea. Strategic planning is nothing more than a process of planning specific strategies to get from one place to another. Business management has had decades of experience with strategic planning, and the process is described in easy-to-understand steps[1] in Chapter 4. It is particularly well-suited to COPC.

A long-range planning process that identifies opportunities and barriers, emphasizes specific strategies, and adapts to a changing environment will help a COPC team focus attention and resources. One of the frustrations of COPC is the seemingly endless list of potential health problems to address, each with numerous possible intervention strategies. In the early stages of the COPC process, all possibilities seem inviting, exciting, and important. But no one can do everything, and you run the risk of diluting your effort if you try to go in too many directions at once.[2] To focus a COPC effort is often a difficult task, unless you take an organized approach to planning and answer the following questions: What's the health problem or question to be addressed? What are the necessary data and how will they be obtained? What might be possible solutions and which of them is most appropriate? Who will perform the tasks?

The COPC process inherently involves establishing priorities or goals, implementing plans, and monitoring results. This type of planning may be foreign to health professionals, many of whom do not have to plan ahead because they have a set schedule that they know will be consumed with patient care. Even if your organization does not ordinarily engage in strategic planning, we advise you to undertake such a process for your COPC efforts. Planning ahead will help your team get involved at all levels, form a consensus about important issues, formulate goals and objectives, and focus on incremental steps or strategies. Since any COPC process involves many steps and perhaps years of work, you must be committed to this dynamic process of planning for the long haul.

3. Community involvement. COPC activities should originate within the community. A team approach that includes working with community members is more likely to sustain a COPC effort and reach a wide population than the health care organization's working alone. Medical practices, hospitals, public health departments, and other organizations that provide health care are usually seen as reputable and trustworthy entities in the community. Health professionals usually enjoy the same level of respect. When these trusted individuals or agencies become involved in community health projects, they help solidify their place in the community. Their involvement can help attract community people to the project and ensure a good beginning. Likewise, if they stop participating, the community may follow suit or even lose trust. Of obvious importance to the community is the belief that health organizations are interested in its problems.

COPC requires networking among professionals, lay groups, agencies, and institutions. Involve yourself actively. This may be an unfamiliar and daunting experience. It is not emphasized in most health professionals' training, but it usually isn't difficult. Being an effective participant in community processes requires time, sensitive listening skills, non-judgmental receptivity, and a willingness to learn new skills. Seek assistance from community organizers who advocate on behalf of health promotion and disease prevention. Being community-based means responding to a community agenda and involving community members as integral members of a team. COPC can mean having to share decisions and give up control. Willingness to invite community input and share control will result in long-term benefits, one of which is the trust a community will develop when its members appreciate your interest and commitment. Chapter 5 provides further discussion.

4. Willingness to quantify. You can't get very far into a COPC process without willingness to gather good, hard numbers and look at them. A com-

EXAMPLE 2.1
Quantifying Problems May Change Approach

Problem Changed from Teen Pregnancy to Lack of Prenatal Care
Tierra Amarilla, New Mexico
Authors: Bill Wiese and Robert Rhyne

A rural, predominantly Hispanic community in New Mexico, Tierra Amarilla, organized a COPC process in 1986. The medical practice in the community, La Clinica del Pueblo, led the effort and was interested in addressing teen pregnancy, which health professionals considered the biggest health problem facing the community.

To characterize the problem, the team abstracted data from birth certificates for the county census divisions that were identified as the practice catchment area. The data revealed that the teen pregnancy rate for the community was actually lower than for the county and the state. They also revealed, much to the surprise of the COPC team, that the level of prenatal care was much lower than for the state as a whole. Therefore, the team changed the problem focus from teen pregnancy to prenatal care among pregnant teens. An important lesson was learned: that providers' impressions of the community's important health problems are not necessarily borne out by objective data.

mon mistake, particularly for clinical providers, is to think that they already know the health problems facing the community. Quantifying a problem is an essential step and often leads to surprising new insight (see Example 2.1).

Quantifying a problem will enable you to track an intervention's impact, positive or negative, and report back to the community. Evidence of impact provides a big boost. "Hey, we changed something in our town; things are better." Even evidence of no impact can provide a boost. Looking at data that you have collected is the reward. It provides an opportunity to reassess strategies and redirect efforts. Quantitative information also helps you evaluate how well a project was executed.

You will need to describe your community or target population in quantitative terms and monitor your use of resources. Data management is usually best done with a computer and will require someone with relevant skills. A good start may reside in the existing office management system for billing, reporting, patient education, or other service needs. It is possible to create a relational database connecting management, clinical, and outcome databases. Database software comes pre-installed on most new computers, and many inexpensive off-the-shelf statistical packages are available. Epi-Info is available free of charge from the Centers for Disease Control and Prevention in Atlanta. (Call the EpiInfo Hotline for Technical Assistance, [404] 728-0545; e-mail: EpiInfo@cdci.cdc.gov.)

Interest in the measurement of outcomes highlights the commonality between community-oriented practice principles and managed care principles. This adds another compelling reason to believe in and work for community-based partnerships that can achieve better health outcomes and reduce costs.

5. Resources. The most tangible prerequisite is the availability of resources, including staff time, space (for work, meetings, file storage, etc.), equipment, access to information, and access to the community. Initiating COPC will draw upon resources, taking time and energy. If available resources are insufficient, however, either the scale of the COPC activities must be reduced or additional resources developed. Ultimately, resources will have to match the scale of your COPC effort and may even determine scale. Take inventory; identify your practical limits.

Resources can be negotiated from community organizations. Help and in-kind assistance can often be found in the local public health system, health councils, educational institutions, and other local provider systems such as hospitals, nursing homes, and home health services. You may find individuals with skills in computer applications, survey design, education/communication, and marketing.

Keep in mind that COPC doesn't always require large amounts of special resources. One physician encouragingly observed, "The only required resource for COPC is your own interest in doing something beyond seeing patients in your office every day!"[3] Small projects, often very useful in getting started in COPC, may require little extra effort and can often be done within existing capabilities. Volunteers can be helpful, particularly with community legwork. Needed data may already be available in municipal, public health, or social agencies.

Although many resources can be found within your organization and community, certain technical assistance and consultant services may need to come from outside sources. The type of assistance needed and availability of appropriate consultants should be discussed as part of strategic planning efforts. For example, do you need a statistician to develop data collection instruments and advise on the analysis of your data? Is there a nearby school of public health with students who might be interested in developing a joint COPC project?

6. Economic impact. Like any undertaking, COPC must be compatible with the organization's long-term economic viability and its objectives for growth. While most people are not attracted to COPC as a way to make money, COPC may become part of an investment strategy to enhance financial viability.

Unfortunately, the traditional fee-for-service reimbursement system penalizes the COPC practitioner because any activity that takes people away from direct patient care also decreases patient revenue.[4,5] Through careful and creative planning, however, COPC interventions that involve delivery of clinical services can be incorporated into the practice as reimbursable services.

Several aspects of the COPC process may directly or indirectly help the organization's ability to plan its economic future and generate revenues, particularly with capitation, managed care, and population-specific health care contracts. Managed care systems can concentrate on population-specific health care concerns and COPC interventions that improve health and may result in reduced costs. Examples of activities that may generate revenues include improved practice planning or outreach to segments of the population not currently seen by the practice; consultative and educational roles; cost-containment activities; generation of grants and contracts; and designing new avenues and systems of health care delivery.

In today's climate of managed care, competitive marketing, and retention of population base (market share), it may be necessary to invest in these activities regardless of your organization's financial status. The investment advances financial viability through program growth and development. Here are some practical benefits:

▶ Improved position to compete for contracts for managed care;

▶ Improved loyalty and stronger client base;

▶ Partnership with other community institutions;

▶ Access to resources, volunteers, grants and contracts;

▶ The opportunity to work with a healthier population.

Not all managed care organizations will give priority to community-oriented goals. This is particularly true for those that are for-profit. Nevertheless, as the public sector assumes responsibility for financing managed care, as in Medicaid managed care, and demands accountability, the organizations will increasingly have to address community and population-wide issues.[6]

OTHER CONDITIONS THAT FAVOR SUCCESS

If your organization meets the basic prerequisites for COPC, look for other conditions that favor success in the COPC process. The condition that most favors success is success itself. Experience is something for which everyone should strive. The more experience you have in the COPC process, the more comfortable you will feel working on a community level and the more success you will have. In this section, we describe other conditions that are helpful (see the checklist in Table 2.2).

1. **Relevance.** Participants in the COPC process will not be enthusiastic unless the process seems pertinent to what they value in their jobs or see as a goal for the practice and community. Projects compatible with managed care principles are particularly relevant. It may require considerable education and/or persuasion to establish a broad sense of relevance, but failure may be the alternative.

2. **Affordability.** A realistic business plan will reveal whether a COPC initiative is affordable. Ultimately, all costs, whether dollar outlays or expen-

---

TABLE 2.2
Checklist of Conditions that Favor Success

1. **Relevance.** Will the proposed activities address problems that are perceived as important?

2. **Affordability.** Will your business plan show that you can cover costs? Can COPC team members devote work time to the COPC effort?

3. **Feasibility.** Will your plan be recognized and accepted by staff and others as feasible and plausible?

4. **Condition of practice.** Will the clinical practice be financially stable? Will its leadership be stable? Does the quality of clinical service allow expansion to a community focus? These should not become issues that interrupt the COPC process.

5. **Staff satisfaction and rewards.** Do all staff understand the rationale and potential value of caring for the community? Will they support a COPC process, whether or not they are directly involved?

6. **Acceptance by peers.** Are you going to get enough positive reinforcement from your peers to keep you going? Will they participate and collaborate?

---

ditures of time, have to be covered from savings, donations, earnings, external revenues, or returns in terms of growth, goodwill, or other future gains. The budget must be monitored and revised as needed. The time that COPC team members devote should come out of work time, not added to an already busy schedule.

3. Feasibility. The COPC project plan must be recognized as feasible and plausible. Written objectives tied to a good management plan can help promote a sense of feasibility. Progress reports to staff with interim measures should be frequent and adequate to verify progress. Participants need to see that the objectives are practical, achievable, and will result in important outcomes.

4. Condition of practice. Only clinical practices or health-related agencies that are alive and well should become involved in a COPC process. Certain imperatives must be attended to before COPC can succeed. These

EXAMPLE 2.2
Empowered Staff Are More Effective

Lunch Meetings Canceled
Stovall, North Carolina
Authors: Robert Rhyne and Tom Koinis

In the rural community of Stovall, North Carolina, the staff of the clinic were excited about starting a COPC process and making an impact on the health of the community. They obtained a small grant, hired a COPC coordinator, and began the process.

The coordinator was given an office in the clinic, and regular meetings were scheduled to plan the process. At lunch times the staff began having meetings to discuss progress and plan strategies.

After a while the staff began to "burn out" on the COPC lunch-time meetings. They felt they had no free time during the day to break from their busy work schedules. Because an open atmosphere had been created and the COPC team frequently evaluated their own process, the staff felt free to air the problem and ask that their lunch times no longer be filled with COPC business meetings. The meetings were changed to a different time, and the participants became much more enthusiastic.

problem. Ideally, this will lead to participation from a variety of community professionals and peers.

SCALE YOUR PROJECT TO AVAILABLE RESOURCES

One of the limiting factors in generating enthusiasm for COPC is the issue of scale. How much is enough? How large should the effort be? Where should we set our sights? The range of activities that involve the community can run from narrowly focused projects addressing short-term situations to broad, long-term undertakings. COPC activities do not have to be "all or nothing." They can evolve a step at a time, focusing initially on smaller projects such as health fairs and building to larger, more involved projects such as reduction of cardiovascular risk factors.[7] Many people

5. Staff satisfaction and rewards. With appropriate involvement in planning, staff will work hard on behalf of COPC because it will enhance their sense of satisfaction and purpose. Most staff want to have an impact on the health of their community. They want to be proud of their organization and be respected as useful in their community. Staff will need to understand why their organization is considering COPC and what their role will be. Talents relevant to COPC, such as data analysis, community organization, and resource development, may previously have gone unappreciated.

Staff also need to understand that they will be given release time to work on COPC and not be expected simply to add to their regular duties. Other staff members also need to be aware what COPC staff are doing so that there is no resentment when they are asked to cover for colleagues working on COPC tasks. Understanding and acceptance by staff are prerequisites to effective involvement and staff satisfaction.

Rewards must be sustaining. A sustained effort will occur only if everyone feels rewarded by the experience. Extra work and overtime must be appropriately acknowledged. A management plan should include regular meetings which allow full participation, recognition of participants' contributions, and support for relevant achievements. Give credit where credit is due.

The COPC process must be fun as well as rewarding in order for everyone to go the long haul. As a leader or manager within an organization, examine your own feelings. A positive attitude starts at the top. It is important to any COPC process that frequent self-evaluation be performed. This can be an informal discussion at the end of meetings on "how are we doing?" and "how is this process going for everyone?" This gives the staff responsibility for the process and empowers them to speak up when something is not right (see Example 2.2). Their continued involvement, enthusiasm, and satisfaction are integral to COPC success.

6. Acceptance by peers. Most professionals will persist in an activity when peer recognition and acceptance are evident. Any project that lies beyond the boundaries of approval from one's professional peers is at risk of being relegated to low priority and eventually dropped. Peer acceptance is accomplished when others value the subject targeted by the COPC effort. Recognize what exists in the professional community and include others in the process who are already working on a particular needs include financial stability, a stable leadership and staff, and a system that provides adequate quality of care.

▶ **Financial stability.** Managers of a new or financially unstable practice will be understandably preoccupied with cutting costs, expanding market share, and generating revenue. When a practice is struggling to survive, community outreach is usually not a high priority, and COPC is unlikely to gain significant attention or support. In contrast, when a practice is financially stable, its focus can turn toward the community and COPC, allowing for allocation of staff and other resources to the COPC effort.

▶ **Stable governance and staff.** COPC takes time. It is crucial to sustain focus and commitment throughout the process. A broad base of interest and support within the governing structure is important, whether the governance resides in a health agency, a clinician-run practice, a board of directors, or a managed care organization. Governance that incorporates community input is particularly well-suited to COPC. Stability and consistency among the leadership and key participants can be critical. Departure of a key COPC team member can compromise the entire effort unless careful planning and documentation have been incorporated into the process. A new person should be able to step in and easily review the process to date. Having an effective administrative structure in place can provide a model.

▶ **Quality of care.** Quality of care for individual patients in a clinical setting must be acceptable. This is an ethical imperative. In accepting responsibility for patient care, give priority to resources that ensure quality. Clinical services of recognized quality will help build credibility and open opportunities in the community. Conversely, if quality is seen as lacking, the community's mistrust will stand as a barrier to the development of COPC.

who are starting out in COPC make an error by setting goals that are far too ambitious or by addressing goals that are unrealistic in terms of time and resources. The COPC process and projects should fit within the capabilities of the health care organization and community. A limited project that succeeds is better than an extensive one that flounders. Early successes will build interest and support as well as experience for taking on bigger projects (see Example 2.3).

Decisions about scale, like other primary planning decisions, should involve all potential participants and include consideration of specific objectives, program options, and resources. A young health care delivery organization may want to begin delving into COPC by identifying a single problem on which to work. The mechanisms established to investigate sub-populations can eventually be the basis for investigating larger problems and populations. Once an organization initiates the process, community resources can be identified and the process can be expanded into the community. A more established practice or agency can begin with a community-based project. Wherever you decide to start, stay within your means and develop the process with adequate planning and forethought.

BUILD ON WHAT ALREADY EXISTS

Every practice or health care setting has its own strengths. To become comfortable with the idea of COPC, identify and build on existing strengths, skills, time and resources, and in particular, existing objectives.

Most health care organizations have service as a principal focus. It is helpful to view the service function of a clinical practice as an interaction between what professionals within the organization already offer and the potential for expanding services to the community. The difference between the two reflects the potential of the practice to become involved in the community. It has implications with respect to the willingness and motivation of a practice to be responsive to priorities in the community and, ultimately, to share decision-making and control.

The organization should have service objectives that allow for flexible time commitments and are compatible with COPC. Those involved in the COPC process use an analytic approach coupled with community involvement to identify needs, implement an intervention, and monitor the result. Those involved should have the energy and time during working hours to participate. Fortunately, the approaches used by many organizations, in-

---

EXAMPLE 2.3
Scale Must Be Appropriate for Early Successes

Trash Lots and Cars (TLC) Project Provides Early Successes
Bowdoin Street Community Health Center, Boston, Massachusetts
Author: Suzanne Cashman

The community advisory board of the Bowdoin Street Health Center
(BSHC) agreed with the center's director and staff on the range of
primary care services to be delivered from the health center's beginning in 1972. Fifteen years later, as the Kellogg Foundation considered funding the Carney Hospital's proposal for an inner-city COPC
demonstration, the health center, under Carney's license, recognized
that it needed to resurrect its original goal. That goal was to provide
a full range of health services that were not only community-based,
but were developed and delivered through a working partnership
with community members. The hospital and health center sought a
reactivation of the grassroots, community-based outlook that had
waned as funding had become more categorical and tied to specified
types of programs. Through the Carney-BSHC-COPC linkage, while
anticipating funding by Kellogg, a student intern working for the
Carney COPC center spent two summer months talking to Bowdoin
Street area community members and local agency leaders. The goal
was to increase the community's awareness of the health center while
cultivating an interest in participating in a community meeting to
identify local health issues.

---

cluding community clinics, managed care organizations, and public health
agencies, are readily adaptable to this process. The busy health professional
who takes the time to learn COPC skills may be able to expand the scope of
service provided by his or her practice and improve the organization's position to attract managed care contracts and health care grants.

REFERENCES
1. Pegels C, Rogers K. Strategic *Management of Hospitals and Health Care Facilities.* Rockville,
    MD: Aspen; 1988.

The intern's efforts culminated in a meeting at the health center in the fall of 1989. About a dozen participants attended, along with the health center director and medical director. The health center staff "already knew" that the major health issue was substance abuse, and while they felt no need to meet, obliged the community members by hosting the meeting. Subsequently, through a series of meetings, residents identified a range of public health problems in the community, and sought common themes. Concern for the breakdown of the family was a recurring theme but represented a problem that participants felt was too sensitive, diffuse, and complicated to address as a first effort.

Consequently, the decision was made to focus on another problem that had been identified through the meetings, one that was concrete and specific — the neighborhood's continuing problems of abandoned cars, broken street lights, empty lots, and trash. Working together, community members and health center staff developed the environmental TLC (Trash, Lots, and Cars) Project. The project was a success and created a nascent partnership between the health center and the community. The project has resulted in regular neighborhood clean-ups as well as a system for reporting abandoned cars, empty lots, and broken street lights. Each of 150 empty lots in the community has been researched, and many have been converted to "tot lots" and community gardens. Residents and businesses continue to work with health center staff not only to maintain these efforts to build a safe, attractive environment, but to work on an array of community health problems.

2. *Healthcare Forum Journal*. May/June 1992; 35.
3. Babitz ME. Doing something is better than doing nothing. In: Nutting PA, ed. *Community-Oriented Primary Care: From Principle to Practice*. Washington, DC: US Department of Health and Human Services, Health Resources and Services Administration; 1987;86-1:23-27.
4. Rogers DE. Community-oriented primary care. *JAMA*. 1982;248:1622-1625.
5. O'Connor P. An opposing view. *J Fam Pract*. 1989;28:206-208.
6. Showstack J, Lurie N, Leatherman S, Fisher E, Inui T. Health of the public: the private-sector challenge. *JAMA*. 1996;276(pt 13):1071-1074.
7. Nutting PA. Community-oriented primary care: the challenge. In: Nutting PA, ed. *Community-Oriented Primary Care: From Principle to Practice*. Washington, DC: US Department of Health and Human Services, Health Resources and Services Administration; 1987;86-1:537-539.

CHAPTER 3

Building a COPC Team

Henry Taylor
Marma McIntee

ABSTRACT

Teams are groups of people pursuing shared goals. COPC teams enable their members to pool diverse skills, tap community resources, and get the work done, but they also require new thinking, and building consensus can be frustrating and tedious. The COPC process requires different teams at different times. Composed of physicians and clinical staff, local leaders, and possibly community activists, the project initiation team begins the process by learning the community's history and health priorities. It then evolves into the implementation team, which plans and implements the COPC process, providing the long-term vision, leadership, and person power. The community advisory board is made up of traditional and non-traditional community leaders who are not on the COPC team, yet are invaluable for rallying community support, maintaining continuity, taking on new programs, and mobilizing volunteers. Partnerships enhance the team's ability to communicate with the community, secure community buy-in, build relationships, gain resources, and develop expertise. Strategic planning, a well-defined mission and roles, community ownership, and communication are all critical to the success of a COPC team.

INTRODUCTION

This chapter discusses how to build and maintain a COPC team. It explores the definition and qualities of teams, their advantages and disadvantages, and techniques of COPC team building.

When planning the type and constitution of your COPC team, consider the following issues:

▶ People. The individuals and their unique energies and skills (do you have the right number?);

▶ Vision. Shared mission, goals, and objectives;

▶ Roles. Job allocation and interpersonal dynamics;

▶ Structure. Systems that allow your team to work as a coordinated unit; and

▶ Partnerships. Affiliations with other community groups.

ADVANTAGES AND DISADVANTAGES OF WORKING IN TEAMS

Teamwork implies joint action on a specific project toward a common goal,[1-3] with some sense of a common vision and unique roles. Teams allow people and groups to pool diverse skills in order to get a job done. Managing and nurturing teams challenges you to bring people together while simultaneously identifying and mediating their differences.

The principle underlying teams is that the whole is greater than the sum of its parts. If you look at the specifics of your situation, many of the components may already be in place. COPC provides the framework to rally a variety of people behind a common cause. For example, local corporate entities can fund COPC efforts and benefit from being advertised as sponsors. Furthermore, building a team with broad representation will put you in touch with many segments of your community, helping you "get the word out." Once team members feel ownership of the process, they can reach much farther into the community than can a single busy health professional, attracting additional volunteers and leaders. They can help facilitate the community's feeling of ownership, and thus bring many more people together to achieve the desired goal.

Often, being in a team works solely because we are in contact with new and different points of view. When a team considers a problem, the solutions that come from brainstorming, discussion, and compromise are usually more creative and rewarding than solutions devised by individuals on their own. Collaborating breeds excitement, and established leaders will further develop their skills by working in the group.

In addition, successful COPC interventions often rely on team members and volunteers to "get the work done" and recruit *other* volunteers. A

TABLE 3.1
Advantages and Disadvantages of a Team

Advantages	Disadvantages
1. Members can share interests and optimize individual effort.	1. A team requires time and effort to initiate and maintain.
2. Community services can be expanded beyond a practice setting.	2. Individuals may feel loss of autonomy.
3. Community awareness can be increased.	3. They may feel that their time schedules have been disrupted.
4. More people can take ownership of the problem and the COPC process.	4. Some may not want to share credit.
5. New people can take on leadership and volunteer roles.	5. Conflicts between team members will arise.
6. Current leaders can learn more about leadership and enhance their abilities.	6. Teamwork takes a lot of time.
7. Collaborating lessens duplication of effort.	7. Roles and responsibilities may become confused.
8. Better services can be provided.	8. Traditional power relationships may change.
9. Participating groups or agencies can gain credibility and visibility.	
10. New clientele can be reached.	
11. The variety of ideas can increase the depth of possibilities.	
12. Many hands make lighter workloads.	

person tackling a COPC project alone may have difficulty finding people to do the work because he or she is the only person with a vested interest.

Other advantages of teams are summarized in Table 3.1, as are disadvantages.[4] As part of a team, you may not always get your way. Understanding a community's point of view may require thinking in new ways. Health professionals are trained to be problem solvers. Community members, on the other hand, may not approach a problem with the analytic rigor developed through formal health education. Intent on a specific goal yet coming from many different walks of life and value systems, they may not see issues the same way.

Building consensus on a difficult issue can be frustrating and tedious. Task-oriented clinicians and administrators may resent the time involved in the group process; they will need to devote special skills and energy to manage interpersonal dynamics.

As a rule, any work using a team approach will take longer than you anticipate. It takes time to consider each member's agenda; however, time spent up front in team building and planning will significantly reduce the time required later to resolve conflicts.

COPC REQUIRES TEAMS FOR GOALS AND PROCESSES

A COPC process requires different teams at different times.[1] At any given time, one will be the principal team moving the process forward. In this book, we refer to it as the "COPC team." Specific types of COPC teams include:

- ▶ Project initiation team

- ▶ Implementation team

- ▶ Community advisory board

- ▶ Volunteer team

- ▶ Partnership

Some teams are goal oriented, develop in response to a specific community health problem, and develop immediate action plans. Process-oriented teams focus on general community development issues and spend more time on group dynamics, needs assessments, and political strategies. Many communities begin with specific interventions addressing an immediate health concern and then develop more extensive community development efforts.

EXAMPLE 3.1
Team Building in COPC

A Variety of Teams for Different Situations
Franklin, West Virginia
Author: Henry Taylor

When Pendleton Community Care began in 1982, it had a clear mission: "Dedicated to improving the health of residents of Pendleton County." This geographic, population-based approach allowed the new clinic to go beyond a disease-oriented clinical practice to develop community based activities. The nine-member governing board had a majority (five) elected by a community membership, with two appointed health experts, the clinic administrator, and a staff-elected representative. The board performed needs assessments and coordinated overall activities. A management team helped coordinate clinical, fiscal, and administrative decisions.

In fiscal year 1991, over half of the corporation's operating budget was in non-clinic programs: COPC, school-based health centers, in-home care of the elderly, a regional adolescent pregnancy specialist, teen natural helpers, worksite wellness programs,

---

Project Initiation Team: Getting The Ball Rolling

COPC processes are often initiated by people working in the health care system, such as a small team from a primary care setting or health agency. That group, the project initiation team, may be composed of clinic staff and physicians, local leaders, or community activists or other volunteers. Key community leaders may be helpful in determining which formal and informal leadership networks may facilitate or impede health improvement efforts. Chapter 5 discusses techniques for identifying these community leaders.

Bear in mind, however, that the team that initiates a COPC process may be different from the one that implements it, because these functions require different skills. Don't be surprised if the composition of the team changes as you move from initiation to implementation. Project initiation team members can go on to serve as advisory board members.

and membership benefits. Most activities were directed at one sub-population (teens, elders, worksites, or members) or one particular issue (adolescent pregnancy, or falls among the elderly). At times, specific community or agency input was required. The most formalized system arose around teen issues. There was a School Health Advisory Council, a natural helpers advisory council, and clinic staff involvement on the school system's Family Life Issues Task Force.

However, not all activities had formalized structures, nor had they always been effective. Turf boundaries between institutions and agencies had been especially hard to overcome. For awhile, the clinic administrator, the director of the nursing home, and the head of the county committee on aging had lunch once a month to discuss elder issues. A change in leadership led to a break in the routine and the group stopped meeting, although all participants said they wanted to continue. After a year and a half of tentative dialogue—and then only in response to the external threat of managed care and the persuasion of the clinic administrator—the clinic board, another clinic's board, and the local board of health joined together to form a larger corporation to help negotiate more favorable contracts than either agency could do alone.

Your project will gain swifter acceptance if you spend time learning about your community's history with other health projects. Maybe the local health department is in Phase II of an APEX/PH (Assessment Protocol for Excellence in Public Health) project. Maybe a PATCH (Planned Approach to Community Health) group was formed, but dissolved when a key facilitator moved away. Hospitals have often done extensive community needs assessments, and they may have advisory committees involved in outreach.

Individuals who have dedicated time and money to their community will want to be involved early in your planning rather than after *you* have decided what they should be doing. Neglect their input, and you may hamper your later success. At the same time, just because they made an unsuccessful attempt to do something several years ago does not mean it will fail again. Community interest could have been stimulated by the initial effort. Interpersonal conflicts may have hampered an otherwise sound project. What counts is whether the project initiation team adequately identifies what went wrong before and incorporates that knowledge as it evolves into the implementation team.

Implementation Team: Long-Term Person Power
The implementation team plans and implements the COPC process, providing the long-term vision, leadership, and person power to accomplish one or more projects. To make this broader team of people work, special effort must be made to establish effective communication among the health system, implementation team and the community. No one sector should automatically assert control throughout the COPC process. The leadership for the team should be identified after it is assembled.

Formation of the implementation team may occur at any stage. However, the earlier the community is involved, the more commitment and ownership they will feel, and the more likely a true team effort will evolve. Involving the community at later stages of the process may develop a "we versus they" split that could lead to the project's downfall. The ultimate decision about timing must be made by the project initiation team.

Community Advisory Board: Leaders Who Ensure Commitment
The community advisory board is useful whenever the COPC project has created a structure that accommodates organized, ongoing participation and vision from community members who are not part of the COPC team. It takes time, effort, and patience to develop, and its role has to be carefully defined and understood. Nonetheless, this advisory team of community leaders—including professionals, civic leaders, public officials, business representatives, school officials, clergy, and the public—is vital to ensuring community commitment and ownership. Its formal structure is distinguished from a mere list of volunteers who are willing to work on various specific projects.

Successful projects usually require both a COPC implementation team and a community advisory board. Many professionals and local leaders— even those imbued with missionary zeal—cannot afford the time, resources, energy, or community-wide commitment to plan and sustain the day-to-day details of the program. The community advisory board provides a solution for those people, serving as a valuable resource even though it may meet infrequently. Members usually enjoy sufficient respect to rally community support and mobilize volunteers. They also can help to ensure the ongoing community participation required to sustain the project, maintain continuity, and take on new programs.

A community advisory board can sometimes seem a cumbersome, volatile, and misdirected means by which to rectify community health problems. Board members may appear to have disparate agendas, political histories that prevent effective cooperation, inaccurate information, or other problems. However, any time lost up front is usually more than made up later as the project swings into high gear.

Include as many community members as possible on the board while keeping the total number to a manageable level of about 10 to 15. The traditional leadership and power structure of the community (e.g., elected officials, business, labor, school representatives, clergy) must be represented. A special effort should be made to involve non-traditional leaders, especially since they often represent groups with higher levels of health needs. Focus groups, community surveys, and similar techniques can be utilized to identify formal and informal community leaders.

Be inclusive and expansive. By inviting all affected groups, chances increase that the project will be viewed as credible and fair. Various individuals and groups will likely float in and out of the project, depending on interest. In the beginning, it may be necessary to start with a nucleus of stalwarts who are committed to you and to the project. Regularly revisit and reflect on board composition – have all the right people been invited?

Pressing local problems, a tradition of community commitment, and/ or dynamic or respected leaders often bring citizens together. It can be tempting, for both the leaders and the followers, to "leave it to the experts," whether they are process experts (e.g., government officials) or content experts (e.g., health professionals). This approach can be a formula for failure because it does not involve the community. The objective is to expand ownership of health problems and the COPC process by incorporating the project initiation team, the implementation team, and the community advisory board in decision-making. The weight carried by each will depend on the issue being addressed.

The community advisory board should provide input and direction, but it should not necessarily be the primary decision-making authority.

The community advisory board should influence how projects are selected and conducted and how project funds are obtained and used, but the COPC team has the job of making the ultimate decisions.

One frequent, salutary by-product of COPC is that new leaders emerge because of their interest in a particular project. The titular leaders of the COPC program should rejoice when this occurs, for it means the community has committed itself to the process. The board needs specific tasks, also. Fundraising is usually near and dear to most community leaders and is a good task for the board. Public relations, networking with parallel projects, and establishing the overall vision are also appropriate activities.

Volunteer Team: Your Front Line

Sometimes, the COPC team may need additional volunteers to carry out a project. This might be a discrete short term activity such as administering a survey or monitoring a booth at a health fair, or it may be a long-term activity such as serving as a weekly visitor to homebound elders. The pool of available volunteers may include local service clubs such as Kiwanis or Rotary Club, high school service clubs such as Key Club or Future Nurses of America, teen religious organizations, or neighborhood associations. These volunteers may not have a personal interest in COPC, and will likely not have decision-making authority (except through a representative who may also serve on the implementation team or community advisory board). Yet they are often your "front line" representatives to the community.

To make their jobs easier and more effective, follow these rules of thumb:

▶ Clearly define specific tasks and reasonable responsibilities.

▶ Train early, often, and well.

▶ Communicate often to prevent misunderstandings. Be open to feedback from volunteers. They may offer valuable insight into public perception of the project and how it can be improved. Give frequent feedback on the project and the volunteers' productivity.

▶ Reassess and reassign as necessary. You may have initially involved them for a specific purpose that didn't work out, but skillful reassignment to other areas can ensure their continued cooperation. Don't hurt their feelings or make them feel inferior; if they are motivated enough to help, you can find a way to use them.

▶ Remind them often, individually and as a group, that you value them.

If you use young volunteers (such as high school students), involve key motivating adults (such as their school advisors). Since your project may be the first community service they have performed, explicit training, close supervision, and an extra dose of patience are necessary.

PARTNERSHIPS: OUTSIDE THE TEAM BUT VALUABLE

According to Webster's Dictionary, a partnership is "close cooperation between parties having specified and joint rights and responsibilities as in a common enterprise."[6] The relationship is not necessarily as close as a team. It is important to make this distinction because people or agencies can become partners of the COPC process without becoming team members.

There are many reasons to form partnerships—to educate, inform, and publicize your efforts to the community and others, thus providing for community buy-in; to build relationships; gain resources; and develop expertise when addressing a health issue exceeding the abilities of any one member.

The project initiation team should seek partners early in the COPC process. Expect to have unexpected groups or agencies express interest in working with your program or the development of your agenda. Explore boundaries of a partnership before making any agreements.[4] All groups in a partnership need to know its purpose, expected duration, short and long term goals, how partners are invited and evaluated, and what is expected of each partner, including specific tasks. Consider an agency's or individual's agenda only as it relates to the goals of the partnership.[7]

As goals are accomplished and direction is refined, new partners may become involved. According to Miller, Rossing and Steele, agencies, organizations, and their representatives form various kinds of relationships.[4] They include:

▶ Pseudo-partnerships (sole ownership). One person or agency dominates the program and others voluntarily assist.

▶ Networks. An informal "keeping in touch." Partners keep each other informed and to some degree can rely on one another when something is needed. They have a stake in the project but are not integral members of the COPC team.

▶ Partial cooperation. Two or more people or agencies cooperate on certain programs or parts of programs. They work separately and retain their independence.

▶ Full partnerships. The program is a joint effort in implementation and overall goals. Most of the decision making, work, and recognition is shared among the partners. A full partnership is a unified team that shares, complements, and extends the participants' abilities and talents. The project initiation team, the implementation team, and the community advisory board are examples.

If we place these partnerships on a continuum we usually gain mutual support as we move toward the full partnership, but we give up individual control and move away from being the sole leaders of the program (Figure 3.1).

"Equal status" may be the single most important element in defining a partnership. When a leader/follower relationship exists, the skills and approaches used to accomplish goals are different. Equal status can be determined by the amount of power, the amount of control, sharing in decisions, sharing contributions, sharing in the workload, sharing the credit, recognition for talents and abilities, and sharing in having ideas heard and accepted by others. In a partnership, all partners contribute equally to the development of goals and making decisions. They are not expected simply to carry out pre-determined decisions. Not every partner will work through every aspect of a decision or project. Partners have certain agreed-

FIGURE 3.1 Dimensions of Involvement

HIGH

▲

Full Partnerships

▶ Mutual planning and execution of long term goals.

▶ Mutual planning and implementation of a program or intervention.

▶ Mutual planning of a program or intervention including assessment, design, training, and evaluation.

▶ Mutual planning of an event with integration of content.

Level of communication, integration, commitment to partnership, and interpersonal skills needed.

Partial Partnerships

▶ Mutual planning of an event with individual segments per partner.

▶ Appearing on a program planned by another partner.

Networks

▶ Mutual scheduling to support each partner.

▶ Mutual scheduling to avoid conflicts with other partners.

▶ Keeping each partner informed of individual activities.

Pseudo-Partnerships

▶ Individual as representative of an agency or organization.

▶ Individual within an agency, organization, or community.

▼

LOW

Adapted from Gibson TL, Moore J, Lueder EJ. *Teamwork in Cooperative Extension Programs.* Unpublished. 1980.

EXAMPLE 3.2
Community Partnerships

A COPC Team Rallies Support
Belleville, Wisconsin
Author: Marma McIntee

The Belleville Community Health Improvement Project (BCHIP) combined representatives from the Belleville school system, the Belleville Family Medical Center, the Village of Belleville, several University of Wisconsin departments, and the University of Wisconsin Cooperative Extension Service; community organizations such as the senior citizens center and church groups; and other individuals with an interest in community health (teenagers, young parents, business representatives, etc.).

As the BCHIP Advisory Council began planning its first project (a community health fair), it was apparent that they would need resources and expertise from other stakeholders and volunteers.

The Council obtained funding from local businesses and health organizations and publicity from the local media, sources not previously involved in BCHIP efforts. Health information and screenings came from an Advisory Council partner, the Belleville Family Medical Center, and other health agencies; facilities were donated by the Belleville school system; volunteers were organized by the Village Clerk and included members of the Senior Citizen Center, the Homemakers Club, the 4-H Club, high school students, and other citizens. In the process, BCHIP created new long-term partnerships and strengthened the community's commitment toward its projects.

upon obligations, and partnerships should identify areas of responsibility in which individuals may act fairly independently.

The goal of COPC is to develop ongoing community/COPC team partnerships, but different individuals and organizations will be active at different times. Some partnerships may result in efforts over long periods to accomplish long-term strategic plans, such as improved healthcare.

Temporary partnerships may be formed to carry out one program goal or activity, such as a community health fair.

Not all prospective partners in the COPC process will have the same interest or willingness to invest time and energy. Partners sign on for a variety of reasons, and while most recognize the value of working together, priorities change. "One of the interesting things about partnerships is that they are dynamic, almost living things... people may come in and leave."[8]

Be aware that there may be potential partners who become involved after the initial partnership formation. Understand their views, even though their representation may not be possible at the time, and even though the partnership may be unable to accept differing points of view.[4] Allowing all potential partners a voice provides the groundwork for community/COPC team partnerships. Potential partners will value the opportunity to have all views heard and responded to, even though they may not be adopted by the partnership. Avoiding such communication could lead to failure and unhealthy competition.

Groups may choose not to join a partnership because of inadequate staffing, difference in program direction or goals, a need to gain internal support before becoming involved, personality differences, etc. These are good reasons not to pursue this partner, but circumstances change over time. Therefore, it is important to "check-in" with reluctant partners during the process and encourage them to become involved. Regardless, keep them informed and retain their support, and their contributions may become more significant as different projects evolve. An open line of communication may avoid blocking efforts by uninvolved entities. Constantly seeking new partners promotes renewal and prevents stagnation in the project, team, or partnership.

ASSEMBLING A TEAM—WHO BELONGS ON THE TEAM?

Health Care Providers: Lending Credibility to the Process

Every clinical practice has experience working as a team, but the physician's role in COPC may be different from the practice setting. Modern medical practices may have large teams of support staff for each physician. In private practice, the physician is the clear leader of the team. In corporate and managed care environments, physicians have had to learn to collaborate with others in order to care for their patients. Likewise, the physicians who become involved in COPC must learn to be team members, not necessarily the team leaders.

The Rural Practice Project[9] of the Robert Wood Johnson Foundation emphasized the overriding importance of project initiation teams in establishing Community Based Health Centers. One or more physicians and an administrator worked together to establish and maintain the practice. Psychological testing, including a Meyers-Briggs Personality Inventory, helped team members find where they best "fit" in the team. While the intent was to build a partnership by establishing governance, in fact, community control was merely a reversal of the power structure seen in private practices. The team, not the physician, made the decisions. Success relied on providers and community leaders sharing leadership.

COPC builds on the physician's experience with teams. Initially, the primary care practice's orientation shifts to an awareness of a "community" outside the office walls. The practice can take leadership in community health activities or participate in activities spearheaded by local health departments and community groups. Mankato, Minn, established an advisory council, linking a broad base of health professionals into a coalition focused on specific community health issues (see Example 3.3) In a successful COPC implementation team, physicians discover that their participation lends important credibility to the process. They help educate non-health professionals about specific health problems. They learn, though, that control of the process is better given to the team as a whole.

Nurses, mid-level practitioners (nurse practitioners and physician assistants), administrators and other clinical support personnel are important contributors to the COPC process.[5] They can serve many functions, from participating on the COPC team, or helping cover the clinical practice while others are involved in COPC activities, to taking major leadership roles. They are usually very familiar with the practice's patients and the issues in the community and are often perceived as less threatening than physicians.

Health professionals need to collaborate actively with community members, convey a clear sense of vision, know their team members, and understand the structures, functions, and processes of the team.

EXAMPLE 3.3
Organizing a Successful Advisory Council

A Local COPC Team Evolves
Mankato, Minnesota
Authors: Linda Hachfeld and Bill Manahan

When Linda Hachfeld, project coordinator, and Bill Manahan, physician director, began characterizing their community and assessing its needs, they first organized a small group of interested representatives from key health organizations: the head of cardiac rehabilitation at the local hospital, the head public health nurse, the director of health services at the local college, the deputy director and grantwriter at the nine-county regional government office, and one other family physician. For the first year, these people comprised the project initiation team, the "Health Action Council," with the chair elected annually.

The group identified alcohol and drug abuse as its initial priority and recruited new members with relevant experience: a school district representative, a lawyer, a community organizer, a parent communication network, and a mental health professional. The group evolved into an implementation team that met monthly for two hours, always on the two physicians' afternoon off. Other members were on salary, which meant the Health Action Council was essentially supported by local organizations. All decisions were made by consensus.

Coordinator: Day-to-Day Task Manager
Central to COPC is the coordinator, who manages the day-to-day organization and tasks of the team. The coordinator should be someone with a working knowledge of health issues and community organization basics. Pay a nurse, social worker, administrator, other health professional, or community person with good management skills to perform this function if possible.

Volunteers: Providing Community Feedback

Volunteers come from many different segments of the community, provide valuable community feedback, and serve as a project's advocates. In almost any community, local service, religious, neighborhood, student, or fraternal organizations will volunteer for worthwhile projects. The main drawback is that volunteers' availability and/or interest may wane, and they may come and go too frequently.

The key to the successful use of volunteers is good training, supervision, reasonable expectations given their background, and a reasonable timeframe. Certificates of appreciation for service help volunteers feel that they are making a meaningful contribution.

Community Participants: Bridging the
Gap Between Community and Professionals

Community members must collaborate actively with the team.[12] They can help gather information, set culturally appropriate priorities, formulate realistic goals, interpret data, and suggest acceptable solutions to problems. Involvement lets citizens learn more about what their health professionals are doing, legitimizes and reinforces community development efforts, and provides advice and support on key health issues.

Certain individuals can be two-way communication channels, articulating the community's concerns to the health professionals as well as translating professional jargon into terms their neighbors understand. Sociologists stress the importance of these "bridging" or "mediation" functions in facilitating community change, whether they occur through individuals or formal and informal social structures. The First International Conference on Primary Health Care in Alma Ata, Soviet Union, in 1978 emphasized the importance of "community health workers." These lay persons with special skills and training in health are important vehicles for dialogue among community, health providers, and policy makers. It helps if these workers keep "one foot in each camp." They need specific, focused training and legitimization by the health system, but they should not become too professionalized ("little doctors").

Other community professionals can help get people to work together. Clergy, social service workers, teachers, politicians, and business representatives formally or informally linked with your COPC activities can provide a succinct summary of needs, reflections on past successes and failures, and innovative suggestions about how to address issues. These "intersectoral" perspectives are especially useful as teams address health problems that have increasingly complex etiologies and solutions.

KEY CONSIDERATIONS IN ORGANIZING TEAMS

When organizing your project initiation team, ask:

▶ What motivates the members?

▶ In the past, how have they best worked together?

▶ What difficulties have they had?

When you determine that other collaborators are needed on the COPC team, ask:

▶ How have previous projects with them succeeded or failed?

▶ Can you or someone else on the project initiation team link effectively with them?

How many community people are on the project initiation team or are potential collaborators on the COPC team? Do they articulate the needs, resources, weaknesses, and strengths of the community? How many are from agencies serving the same target population as yours? Have they been effective advocates, professionals, or case managers?

Try to identify the people who will continue on the COPC team over a long period. At team meetings, review the team's composition. File your notes so you can refer to them as you evaluate and modify your project.

Once your project is off the ground, draw an organizational chart showing the various teams and how they relate to one another. Ask:

▶ What is each person's role?

▶ Who answers to whom on each team? Are lines of authority clear?

▶ Should anyone be added to the teams to provide needed skills?

▶ Can you spot potential role conflicts?

▶ Do team members recognize the multiple roles of others (particularly in small institutions)?

▶ What training is needed? More broadly, what skills need to be developed within your institution? In other key agencies serving the same target population? In patients served by the practice?

FOCUSING A TEAM

Strategic Planning — Shared Vision and Unique Roles

Why discuss strategic planning in a chapter on team building? Because:

▶ You will need your team's input into the planning process.

▶ Your team needs to develop the plan together so they "own" it.

▶ You will need to get consensus on the steps of the action plan and its time frame.

You may be asked to explain and justify your actions to potentially hostile people. Community-Oriented Primary Care is fundamentally a strategic planning process that can sharpen and maintain the focus of your team by developing a common purpose and vision.

If everyone on the team reaches consensus on the goals and expected outcomes of the project, they are much more likely to work together to reach those goals. Try building a consensus on what will be happening with the health of your community three to five years from now. What specifically do you want to accomplish? Why are you going to this trouble?

Since our actions result from our experiences, a "futuring" exercise will help your team break out of their current limitations and imagine a coherent future. Then the team can identify the critical "next steps" necessary to making that future a reality.

Constructing a team mission statement early in the process will focus your team and prepare you for later problems. Members need to discuss where they are going (vision and needs assessment); how they are to get there, including specific tasks (action plans and interventions); how they can work together, playing to the strengths of individual team members (roles); and how they will measure progress towards mutually defined goals (outcomes and evaluation). Strategic planning is discussed more in Chapter 4.

Many think strategic planning is a "linear" process, where you start from one point and move in sequential steps to another. However, COPC requires a more dynamic, process-oriented approach. Rarely do you start from scratch, and usually, other community groups will have tried to improve health before you came into the picture. As we discussed in Chapter 1, the five steps of COPC rarely proceed in sequence. This also means that planning is non-linear; there are multiple feedback loops, and like any real-life situation, constant change is the rule.

A long range strategic planning process should accommodate changing situations and maintain a shared vision. Dr. Jack Bryant has likened improving a community's health to "trying to change a tire while the car is moving."[13]

Teamwork: What Does the Team as a Whole Have to Do to Get a Job Done?

When organizing the team, consider the four phases of each task:[10]

1. **Initiation:** Define the task. Some people are good at articulating the task and what its results should be. These people may not be the best to follow through on details.

2. **Ideation:** Some people easily generate alternative solutions, or know what has worked in the past.

3. **Elaboration:** After the overall approach has been determined, develop specific action plans: the people, time, money, and physical resources required.

4. **Completion:** Select a plan, establish monitoring systems, and get the job done on time and within budget.

**Team Roles: What Do Individual COPC
Team Members Have to Do to Get a Job Done?**
In organizing teams to work with the community, play to the strengths of
your people—assign members according to their interests, competence,
and confidence. However, don't rule out the possibility of assigning someone to a new area. If some tasks do not come naturally to people, allow
them extra attention, time, and space.

There are eight essential roles on any team.

1. **Leader:** Identifies the task and motivates others.

2. **Moderator:** Identifies people to work on tasks and gets
   them involved.

3. **Creator:** Generates solutions, including alternatives.

4. **Innovator:** Locates resources and identifies ways to use
   them.

5. **Manager:** Develops plans to utilize people and resolves
   conflicts.

6. **Organizer:** Organizes time, money, and physical resources.

7. **Evaluator:** Analyzes the alternatives, plans, and results.

8. **Finisher:** Follows through on details to ensure completion.

The roles may be played by different individuals who have different com-
binations of capabilities.[11] In small projects, one person may assume multiple roles.

MANAGING A PROJECT INITIATION TEAM

The project initiation team needs to make the vision and assignment clear
to the implementation team. The initiation team also needs to pay attention to interpersonal relationships and establish effective methods for communication. Initiation team members may continue to provide oversight
and guidance throughout the project.

Charging an Implementation Team

Components of a Team Charter

Table 3.2 provides a template for a team charter. A team charter helps the implementation team know precisely what the initiation team expects. In large bureaucracies or contentious situations, the charter focuses the team, sets boundaries, and is a useful tool for communicating the project to others. It helps identify necessary people, money, and other resources.

The template charter evolved from several years of experience implementing a total quality management process in the West Virginia state government through the "INSPIRE" project; it was refined by the Quality Council of the West Virginia Bureau for Public Health.

TABLE 3.2
Template for a Team Charter

Team Name: _____ Date: _____

Mission: Goals and expected outcomes.

Accountability: Community defined and characterized. Specific need to be addressed.

Boundaries and Constraints: What should not be studied? What decisions can the team make? Can it set its own budget?

Resources: Support services. Budget under the team's control. Available experts. Time and energy the team can put into the project.

History: Brief summary, including project initiation team's discussions in creating the implementation team as well as needs assessments and other activities in the larger COPC effort.

Timeline: Target completion date and intermediate reporting requirements.

Team Representation: Bring together individuals who would work well together as a team. Determine whether each person has the knowledge, skills, time, and influence required to participate effectively on the team.

It's up to you to create a clear statement of the mission, resources, timeline, and expected "deliverables" so that team members can concentrate on the product and meeting deadlines. Write down a brief history of the problem so they can understand its context. Use a project notebook with meeting minutes and progress summaries to keep from reinventing the wheel.

Charging a Team

Drafting a final team charter may take time as the initiation team struggles with characterizing the community and defining the problem. Discussions about interventions may spawn a subgroup that becomes the implementation team, a process that may be more or less formalized depending on the situation.

Once a draft charter is written, team members need to be recruited. At the meetings, develop group cohesion, then thoroughly review the draft charter, checking for clarity and specificity. You may want to retain one or two members of the initiation team on the implementation team, especially until its members become comfortable revising the charter and working as a group.

Communication within the Team

"A team is a small-scale social system and thus must maintain good communication between its members."[13]

Teams are often created in response to external forces: to satisfy a granting agency or legal mandate at the request of local physicians, by non-profit boards in the community, by civic clubs, or as a special problem-focused task force. Your institution's management style may influence who must be a part of the team. Some institutions have existing teams that function well together in other endeavors, but they may not be flexible or innovative enough to switch to Community-Oriented Primary Care. Building new teams, however, requires a significant investment in group process. Understanding your team's history will allow you to respond to future threats and opportunities.

Once a team is formed, many problems can arise. Example 3.4 illustrates what can happen when leaders fail to outline mission, plans, and roles from the beginning. Difficulties also occur when people are thrust into new roles or when organizational changes alter job descriptions.[11] Turf battles and other conflicts can be avoided when team members recognize that every member brings unique talents to the mix. Chapter 4 discusses conflict resolution in more detail.

To prevent destructive gossip and mediate differences, always maintain communication within the team. Communication can be direct, through meetings or one-on-one discussions, or indirect, through e-mail, memos, or newsletters. Meetings can be stifling if not planned carefully. See Chapter 4 for tips on conducting regular, productive meetings.

EXAMPLE 3.4
Conflict in Leadership Roles

Conflict Leads to Meltdown in a Rural COPC Practice
Stovall, North Carolina
Authors: Tom Koinis and Robert Rhyne

The clinic was started almost 20 years ago by two mid-level providers, a husband and wife team. The female member of the team, a clinic nurse practitioner, was the informal leader of the clinic although she never thought of herself in that light. Nevertheless, when things happened in the clinic, it was generally due to her energy and decisions. With a history of providing excellent clinical care, and with the intent of expanding their practice to address some community health issues, the two providers submitted a grant application and were funded to do a COPC project.

In the grant, the nurse practitioner and the clinic's supervising physician were named as co-leaders of the COPC project. The physician's wife, a pediatric nurse, was hired as part-time COPC Coordinator. Because the nurse practitioner felt she already had an good understanding of the COPC process and did not require any additional training, the COPC Coordinator and her physician husband both agreed to attend a COPC training seminar sponsored by the

Continued on the following page.

Continued from the previous page.

granting agency. The training was very experiential, using case studies and small group problem solving to convey factual theory as well
as shaping individual attitudes.

On returning home, everyone was eager to get a COPC process
underway but, given the differences in how each had been exposed
to COPC, the nurse practitioner and COPC Coordinator had different views of the steps involved in the COPC process. Both hesitated,
unsure of how to work together given their differing views on how
to approach the process and who would function as its leader. The
supervising physician held back from leadership, wanting the community to take charge.

As the project progressed, conflict grew between the nurse practitioner and COPC Coordinator because of differences in leadership
style and lack of regular communications between the two. Leadership roles and responsibilities were not clarified, and the growing
conflict led to the eventual resignation of the COPC Coordinator and
the exodus of both mid-level providers from the clinic which they
had founded. The physician was left to continue the work of the selected COPC project but was severely hampered by the loss of not
only his core COPC team members, but his primary health care provider staff as well.

In retrospect, the team could have spent more time getting all leaders to the same point of understanding about the Community-Oriented Primary Care process. Problems in team dynamics should have
been addressed as soon as they arose, determining where the strengths
of individuals lay and where weaknesses existed. The lines of communication among the team's leadership should have been established
early in the process. This leadership team learned that Community-
Oriented Primary Care proceeds at a different and more intense level
of interpersonal involvement than running a practice. The team could
have sought outside help from a variety of consultants or local leaders, although it is often difficult to perceive the problems early in the
process. While objectivity is hard to achieve when viewed from within
the circle, as a group they could have recognized sooner that their assigned roles were different from the roles they were actually fulfilling.

REFERENCES

1. Abramson JH, Kark SL. Community oriented primary care: meaning and scope. In: Conner E, Mullan F, eds. *Community Oriented Primary Care: New Directions for Health Service Delivery*. Washington, DC: National Academy Press; 1983;21-59.

2. Paul B, ed. *Health, Culture and Community*. New York, NY: Russell Sage Foundation; 1955;20.

3. Geiger J. The meaning of community oriented primary care in the American context. In: Conner E, Mullan F, eds. *Community Oriented Primary Care: New Directions for Health Service Delivery*. Washington, DC: National Academy Press; 1983;70.

4. Miller LC, Rossing BE, Steele SM. *Partnerships: Shared Leadership Among Stakeholders*; unpublished. 1990.

5. Kark SL. *The Practice of Community-Oriented Primary Health Care*. New York, NY: Appleton-Century-Crofts;1981.

6. *Webster's Ninth New Collegiate Dictionary*. Springfield, Mass: Merriam-Webster, Inc; 1983;859.

7. Gibson PL, Moore J, Lueder EJ. *Teamwork in Cooperative Extension Programs*; unpublished. 1980.

8. Lamb G. *Extension Agents Offer Guidelines for Building Community Partnerships* [videotape].1989.

9. Madison D. *Starting Out in Rural Practice: The Rural Practice Project - Report of the Director*. Chapel Hill: Department of Social and Administrative Medicine, School of Medicine, University of North Carolina at Chapel Hill; 1980.

10. Mumma F. *What makes your team tick? — Team Work and Team Roles*. King of Prussia, Penn: Organization Design and Development Inc; 1994.

11. Work of Benne, Sheats, Bales, Strodtbeck, Belbin. Cited by: Mumma, F. *What makes your team tick? — Team Work and Team Roles*. King of Prussia, Penn: Organization Design and Development Inc; 1994.

12. Hatch J, Eng E. Health Worker Roles in Community Oriented Primary Care. In: Conner E, Mullan F. *Community Oriented Primary Care: New Directions for Health Service Delivery*. Washington, DC: National Academy Press; 1983;138-166.

13. Bryant J. Personal Communication. September 1991.

CHAPTER 4

Leadership and Management in COPC

Richard Bogue

Richard Roberts

Martin Hickey

> *The final test of a leader is that he or she leaves behind in others the*
> *conviction and the will to carry on.... The genius of a good leader is to*
> *leave behind a situation which common sense, without the grace of*
> *genius, can deal with successfully.*
>
> *—Walter Lippman*

ABSTRACT

The COPC process has varied requirements for leadership and management. In the early stages, COPC leaders articulate a vision and determine the direction the group will take. Later, as managers, they implement decisions moving the group in that direction. Leaders, like managers, have authority because a group confers it upon them. COPC leaders motivate the group by communicating their vision and keeping people focused; by imbuing the project with values that ensure commitment; by creating an environment for personal development and empowering participants; and by exemplifying positive leadership behavior. As managers, they set priorities and recognize limitations; establish a measurable goal and appropriate interventions; and evaluate progress. In order to succeed, both leaders and managers must engage in strategic planning, establish consensus for major decisions, and resolve conflicts by concentrating on the issues and collaborating, especially through well-run meetings. Sharing management responsibilities by partnering with managed care companies—which may save money by keeping their populations healthier—can supply the financial incentives and resources to address community health.

INTRODUCTION

Community-Oriented Primary Care centers on changes in behavior, difficult changes to effect. In the abstract, almost everyone would agree that it is a good idea to institute changes that improve health and well-being. But good ideas remain only good ideas without an organizational structure, a plan, and a system of accountability. This is where the need for effective leadership and good management arises.

Leadership and management—excellence or poverty in these can advance or ruin any effort. They are among the most discussed concepts we encounter. The approaches people take as they lead or manage often seem to be as diverse as the people themselves. Daily experiences show us ineffective, as well as superb, leadership and management skills. Unfortunately, most health professionals do not learn these skills in their educational programs. This chapter strives to stimulate excellence in leadership and management for COPC by describing the differences between the two, the basics of each, and ways to lead and manage in the context of COPC.

AUTHORITY: THE BASIS OF LEADERSHIP AND MANAGEMENT

We can understand the concepts of leadership and management better if we differentiate between them. But first, we can appreciate how they are similar by understanding the concept of authority. Purposeful, organized human behavior occurs in social contexts. In social groupings of all kinds, hierarchies of authority operate. Whether in our family, our workplace, our place of worship, or at an informal gathering of friends, one or another of us exercises more authority than others over certain decisions and how they are implemented. In other words, for any given decision, one of us has more influence over what the group does than others. With this in mind, Max Weber outlines three kinds of authority.[1]

The first is *traditional authority,* in which decisions are justified on the basis of tradition or habit. The power of kings and queens, for example, was viewed as legitimate because their fathers or mothers had held power and "God had ordained it to be thus." The second type is *bureaucratic* or *rational-legal authority.* Here, authority is ascribed on the basis of position in a bureaucracy. A supervisor enjoys rational-legal authority over a subordinate, for example. The third type Weber termed *charismatic authority*. It depends on people following a person's decisions or directions because they are persuaded to do so.

The most important thing to notice about these types of authority is what they have in common. Authority depends on a group of people granting or giving it to someone else. *Authority is not taken by the person who has it. It is given by the people who do not have it to the people who have it.* Even in social contexts, leadership and management are forms of authority that are given by the group to the individual. The citizens respect the governor. The soldiers obey the general. The workers follow the boss.

An individual's authority also depends on the stage of decision-making. A board may set a policy, which is implemented by a CEO, while a department manager may be the principal decision maker in the implementation. Each of these people exercises authority over some phase of group action.

Often, we obscure the details of leadership and management by interpreting group action in terms of a leader and followers, regardless of how many people have authority and may have acted on a certain decision. Largely because it enables us to organize our complex social experiences more easily, we typically attribute group actions—successes and failures—to an individual. Eleanor Roosevelt was referring to millions of people exercising authority over all kinds of decisions and actions when she said, "A leader may chart the way, may point out the road to lasting peace, but many leaders and many peoples must do the building."

LEADERSHIP AND MANAGEMENT

Leadership and management are similar in that they both reflect the authority given by the group to an individual, but they differ in that they occur in two distinctly different phases of group action. Leadership determines what actions the group will take. Management determines how to take them and sees that they're taken. Leadership sets directions for the future, using yesterday and today as guides. Management oversees the activities of today and reviews those of yesterday, using the future direction as a guide. As an example, the COPC team provides the leadership in developing the goal of decreasing the rate of teen pregnancies in a community, and designing an intervention step that offers alcohol-free weekend night dances to the teens. A management subcommittee is formed that has the responsibility of planning, organizing, and conducting the dances.

One person may lead *and* manage a given line of action. It is typical, though, for many people to contribute, with some providing more leadership at one time than another and others carrying out more of the management. COPC magnifies opportunities for both leadership and management because it relies on voluntary collaboration by people from different backgrounds working together as one group on the five phases (or steps). COPC permits, even demands, that different individuals exercise relatively more authority than others at different phases in the process. As a collaborative, community-driven, multi-step, and iterative process, it presents rich opportunities for many people to practice the skills of leadership and management.

LEADERSHIP

The key point for leaders to understand is that they are the catalysts in motivating themselves and other people.[2,3,4] Leaders discover what motivates the group and then show ways to stimulate those motivations. There are five basic elements to creating such a motivating environment: vision, values, personal development, empowerment, and leadership behavior.

Vision

By painting a picture of how things could and should be in the future, a vision connects people's daily efforts to the efforts of their co-workers and team members, to a purpose that is larger than self and more enduring than this quarter or this year. A vision gives a deep, abiding and long-term purpose to group behavior and, therefore, it is the key to excellent leadership. The person who is held by the group as the authority behind a vision has captured the essence of leadership. A good leader helps his or her team keep focused on the vision and how today's activities relate to that vision. How profoundly a vision affects people depends chiefly on the effective use of the remaining elements of leadership.

Values

People give their time, effort, and money to a program, and lend legitimacy to a program's leadership because they believe their investments will advance something of value. If people do not feel the COPC project addresses a value they embrace, there will be little motivation to work for the project.

The COPC team can gain an understanding of the community and health values held by individuals (e.g., a drug-free community for children or a smoke-free indoor environment) through discussions, focus groups, and questionnaires (see Chapter 5 for details). Imbuing the vision, mission, and goals of the project with these values enables people to make personal commitments.

Personal Development

Personal development can occur in many ways. Participation in a community effort can promote learning new skills and new knowledge, which can then be used in other projects or professional work. It can also provide the opportunity to make new friends, create an opportunity to model positive social behavior for one's children or professional apprentices, and meet the basic human need for hope—for being part of something larger than oneself. Finally, it can provide positive exposure to group members who are your potential clients, customers or employers. These values are simple and intuitive and can be communicated clearly to potential team members and volunteers. Leadership, setting the stage for action, includes creating an environment in which personal value and worth can be enhanced.

Empowerment

Empowerment is fundamental to excellence in complex human endeavors. During the Cold War, NATO strategists in Europe estimated that NATO needed far fewer troops than the Soviet Union because, among other reasons, even the smallest NATO units were prepared to act independently. Empowerment to decide and act locally instead of waiting for orders from above was specifically identified as a major advantage, a key to excellence. In COPC and other efforts in which people serve as stewards of the community's well-being, authority in both forms (leadership and management) should be delegated widely.

Enabling others to exercise authority can be very difficult for many leaders and managers, especially if they are professionals who think of themselves as "the experts." Health professionals sometimes have difficulty trusting a lay group to make informed decisions about health.

The blinders of expertness are among the most common and difficult barriers to community health improvement. Relying on expert knowledge often leads to misdiagnosis of community problems, mismanagement of community efforts, and an inability to create a vision toward which people want to work. Example 4.1 illustrates how this can happen quite innocently.

The challenge of empowerment is to establish a system of making decisions that includes everyone from the outset. People will understand limitations: that everyone simply cannot be informed all at once, that not everyone will show up at early meetings, that a smaller group invariably has to initiate the effort before larger groups can be engaged, and that it is prohibitively expensive to interview every member of a community. But when many people are involved in team formation and decision making, the message is that individual input and worth are valued. With motivated followers, an initial leadership group can give up progressively more decision making authority and can nurture leadership behavior on the part of more team members.

Leadership Behavior

Skilled leadership evokes a positive overall atmosphere. Leadership recognizes and makes use of moments of crisis to help motivate, too. Indeed, more than one successful community effort has been launched by a local tragedy. But without a positive overall atmosphere, using crises to motivate creates a stream of emotionally draining experiences, and the motivation wanes when the crisis is over.

A leader's behavior sets the tone as well as the direction and encourages actions that lead to success or failure. When the tone is critical and negative, most of us tend to withdraw or become defensive. When negative comments are made on a regular basis, the effort will fail. The inept "leader" will be left with no one willing to give him or her authority for decision making and no assistance.

Explicitly valuing others' contributions, even when you point out that you do not agree, will go a long way in fostering hard work and commitment by team members. Have faith in, and employ, the COPC team's vision and collective wisdom to keep things on track when people express themselves poorly or offer ideas that strike you as off-base. Never belittle anyone. If you employ consensus-based decision making and yet fail to dislodge an idea that you think is wrong, seriously explore the ways in

EXAMPLE 4.1
Leadership and Empowerment

The Expert Approaches the Community
Philadelphia, Pennsylvania
Author: Richard Bogue

A young researcher stood before a coalition of community groups in Philadelphia several years ago, proposing a community health assessment. He explained that the survey had been designed by experts in the nearby university. It would produce the knowledge needed to show all the community groups present how they could better work together in meeting the city's higher priority health problems. Everyone listened politely. When the researcher was sure he had explained adequately why the survey design was valid and how the information gathering and reporting processes would produce rigorous and accurate results, he asked if anyone had questions. There was a pause and then several people around the room rose from their seats. One person after another assertively informed the researcher that no one in that room, nor anyone in the groups they represented, would participate in "another damned survey." First, they and others had to be in on the project's development from the beginning. And then they had to be assured they could honestly tell their neighbors that they would see benefit from participation. Do these things first, they said, and then we can work with some experts on designing a survey.

After the meeting, a community organizer took the researcher aside and explained that she and the others wanted to work with the university. "But time after time," she said, "researchers come in, do their studies, and disappear, leaving the people with the same problems as before. We're just asking you to worry as much about how to work with us to improve our lives, as you do about the validity of the surveys."

A few months later, a team from the university sat down with community organizers to explore how they could develop a joint grant proposal that would focus as much on community solutions as on survey design.

which *you* may be wrong. Be open to new suggestions. Chances are that this will help you free yourself from seeing the issue in terms of right or wrong. If you still cannot see the wisdom in an idea that gets momentum within the group, consider a modest role for yourself in that part of the group's efforts, and seek other parts of the joint work in which to invest yourself. Henry Miller once observed that "the real leader has no need to lead, [but] is content to point the way."

Following are some specific tips on being a good leader:

▶ Ensure inclusiveness. Partnership comes first, then vision, then planning, then action.

▶ Keep the vision alive. Refer to it frequently. Put a crisp vision statement on a poster board or a transparency and display it at the beginning of every meeting. See if a local printer will donate business cards for project participants that include the vision statement on the back.

▶ As team members become more engaged in COPC, delegate decisions and tasks.

▶ Listen without judging. Learn what each participant seeks. Once it is clearer what motivates people, you can help each individual and the group recognize good matches between individual desires and group objectives. What assignments best fit each aspiring leader?

▶ Remove any professional blinders. Your special knowledge as a health care professional is indispensable, but so are the talents of other team members. Honor their knowledge and experience.

▶ Create an openly positive environment. Make a point of saying so when someone's words or deeds trigger excitement, help you see a problem in a new way, or make your duties run more smoothly.

If there is one consistent theme about leadership from collaborative community health improvement projects like COPC, it is that leadership roles change hands often. People move out of town, serve their term as leader and turn it over to someone else, take on more responsibility in their jobs, or declare victory and call it quits after a particularly gratifying success. Projects that consciously develop new leadership by delegating responsibility and authority go on to achieve additional successes. They provide more community exposure and praise to more volunteers and create more opportunities for additional team members to lead and manage. Excellent leadership actively nurtures leadership by others, trains them, gets out of their way, and is not threatened by their success.

MANAGEMENT

It is the well-managed team that will achieve the ultimate goal of community change in COPC.[5,6,7] Leadership creates the vision and commitment to act. Management provides the operational structures. Below are leadership and management skills that are particularly important for COPC.

Setting Priorities and Recognizing Limitations

While it may be appropriate as a vision, eliminating all unhealthy behaviors in the community cannot be achieved by any COPC team in a foreseeable future. Priorities have to be established. Your team's resources place important constraints on prioritization. COPC is still rarely seen as a mainline business venture, which means that the most valuable resource in a COPC project is people's time. When health professionals participate, they often view their COPC time as lost opportunity costs for their "real" business. However, this may change as more health professionals explore the business potential of COPC in a managed care world.

Material resources never seem to be in adequate supply for collaborative community health improvement efforts, but much can be accomplished with minimal direct funding. In most communities, volunteers and material assistance can be obtained from interested businesses.

Larger foundations, foundations with a national scope of interest, and government agencies are also possibilities. They want to see evidence of accomplishments and support the development of tools and techniques that could help other communities. Local and corporate foundations, on the other hand, often prefer to support direct, local service delivery.

But there are important, and sometimes overlooked, limits to external funding. Grants run out. Fund raising requires investment of time and effort at the expense of other activities. Do not invest effort seeking funds for work that does not fit your vision and plan. This is typically wasted effort and almost always detracts from your goals.

Planning as a Partnership for COPC

With a clear understanding of your limitations, your team can start a long-term planning process to command more resources.[8,9,10,11]

Planning is a process that analyzes the present and the future in order to align near-term activities with longer-term goals. Incorporating such a process helps the COPC team approach problems in an organized manner, anticipate barriers to successful implementation, and maximize input into strategies. Once an ongoing cycle of planning is established, the management structure sustains the collaborative efforts of the organizations and individuals involved in the COPC process.

The classic steps of planning are to establish a purpose or mission, assess the environment, establish a measurable goal and interventions, and evaluate progress. A preliminary assessment of readiness can help a COPC team shore up weak points and evaluate the potential for success. In essence, it examines a community's access to the necessary tools, people, institutions, and resources to undertake a COPC program and starts the partnership building process. Some elements of this initial assessment include:

1. Commitment of initial leadership. A small group (four to six members) must be committed to providing leadership during start-up and planning. We recommend that the COPC project initiation team (see Chapter 3 for additional discussion) represent at least the management and boards(s) of health care organizations, the public health department, and members of the medical community. Participation by these organizations up front is particularly important since a successful COPC effort may change their ongoing operations and may reallocate resources among them. The project initiation team may emerge from an educational COPC cluster committee (described in Chapter 10), a medical practice, a task force in the public health department, or from any number of other sources. Project initiation team members often come from committees that recently completed other community health projects.

The first step of the COPC project initiation team is to (a) clearly express their availability and commitment and (b) designate a chairperson.

The second step is to design a process to develop its membership. One method for developing a larger group is for each project initiation team member to contact three candidates, based on agreed-upon criteria, each of whom in turn is asked to contact three. These contacts can pose questions that are useful in other parts of the planning task force's work, as described below.

No matter how people are identified for participation in the larger group, be certain that they represent the diversity of the community as much as possible. (See Chapter 5 for techniques.) Dimensions of diversity include ethnicity, language, gender, organizational affiliation, type and level of formal training, as well as location. Community projects that start by excluding groups of people are absolutely doomed: even if they succeed as projects, they are not community projects.

2.   **Assess possibilities for expanding the COPC partnership.** Design a written survey or telephone interview which elicits values and attitudes related to a community-responsive or COPC process. Present the results in a project initiation team meeting that is attended by the new, larger pool of possible participants to explain COPC and evaluate it. Maximize enthusiasm by eliciting the group's ideas and promoting the sense of "being there at the first step" through active participation. This approach requires exceptional interaction planning and group facilitation skills (see Chapter 5). It also requires a lengthy meeting, often a half- or full-day summit.

Consider inviting a respected, skilled, and neutral facilitator from outside the local health care community (perhaps from city government, a college, or another community, or a paid group process facilitator). The facilitator's main interest should be in group process, not in the future of COPC. At this first larger meeting no common vision can be presumed, and many of the ideas may be new to many participants. Hence, the potential for a confusing or even acrimonious meeting is high.

3.   **Assess the community's organizational preparedness for planning.** How do people and organizations in your community function? There are probably as many barriers to a community's preparedness for planning as there are organizations and communities. After introducing the larger group to COPC, the project initiation team should do the following:

a. Examine the functioning of local boards to identify connected community leaders. Which boards play an active role in setting long-term plans for organizations that are to partner through COPC? Do the board members take advantage of opportunities to become more informed about health care issues, both locally and nationally? Which individuals serve on the boards of more than one organization that the project initiation team considers a stakeholder in COPC?

b. Identify and utilize people who run especially effective meetings. Whose meetings include healthy debate but also arrive at clear decisions? For whose meetings is follow-up quick and responsive?

c. Identify and model effective management practices. Which management teams are considered proficient? How do they maintain clarity about roles and responsibilities? How do they ensure open communication across organizational units and levels of hierarchy?

d. Examine the functioning of the health care community. What alliances and conflicts exist? How do local providers' affiliations with outside organizations enable or constrain their participation? Does the project initiation team adequately recognize the time and energy already invested by physicians and other caregivers?

e. Identify models of effective conflict resolution in the health care community. How are major conflicts handled? What groups or individuals are especially able to focus on mutual goals rather than past events, personalities, or current barriers? What groups and individuals are most effective at making their goals clearly known?

f. Gain a broad understanding of who comprises the community. What ethnic groups, towns or neighborhoods, and organizations or agencies make up the community? For now, the objective is to ensure inclusiveness (see Chapter 6). Use your findings to design a COPC team. A membership of 10 to 12 approaches the upper limits for highly interactive small group discussion. But the group can be much larger if enthusiasm is wide and strong and someone can lead the group productively. Consider creating other opportunities for active leadership roles, such as task forces, an advisory board, and a volunteer team. (Chapter 3 provides details.)

THE PLANNING PROCESS (STRATEGIC PLANNING)

The full COPC team should participate in answering the following questions, which are outlined in 10 steps below (see Table 4.1). Strategic planning may take a few meetings, as the project initiation team evolves into a larger COPC team.

Step 1 - What values does the group hold with regard to COPC? The values should be as specific as possible. Include values about how the COPC team operates, for example, with consensus, interpersonal respect, teamwork, and integrity. In general, three to seven guiding values will work, and more than 10 or so will water down the agreement. Examples:

> PREVENTION: Our COPC efforts will be aimed at unhealthy behaviors which lead to disease. We believe that preventing disease is better than treating preventable disease after it develops.

> CONSENSUS: our COPC process will engage the opinion of every active team member and work to develop their buy-in. We will attempt to reach consensus on all issues.

Step 2 - Who are the team's communities? A COPC process cannot be all things to all people. Assign priorities. Knowing the prime beneficiaries will make establishing a mission and goals much easier. Refer back to the values and initial assessment. Identify in writing the community you seek to serve; identify a community denominator for use in analyzing health and performance goals. Is the community the county, the town, a neighborhood?

TABLE 4.1
Strategic Planning Steps

STEPS	DEFINITIONS
1. Assess values	Statements of how COPC team will operate, areas of emphasis, and other guiding principles.
2. Identify community	Profile of individuals or groups you seek to serve.
3. Visualize health care	How you think health care will "look" in the future.
4. Develop vision	What you envision for the future health of your community.
5. Determine mission	Purpose and composition of team, what will be achieved, for whom.
6. Develop goals	Broad statement of short and long-range expected accomplishments, the at-risk subpopulation, and the expected change.
7. Define objectives	Action steps, or tasks, necessary to reach goals, responsible person(s), and timeline.
8. Develop strategies and activities	Specific tasks to implement intervention, the number of participants, the outcome measures, the analysis plans.
9. Evaluate performance	Progress in implementing plan, intervention, and evaluation.
10. Seek sustainability	Revisions in strategic plan to incorporate activities in the community health system.

Should more than one community be included? (Chapter 6 discusses community denominators.)

Step 3 - What will the future health care environment look like? Will new health problems arise based on the community's changing demographics? Is there legislation pending that may change the nature or size of a community problem? Will new health care businesses be coming to the community? What is the penetration of managed care? Based on current trends and what is happening in other similar communities, how will your COPC effort respond?

Step 4 - The vision: what should the future be like for our community? Based on the previous three steps, what does the COPC team want to see happening in the community five or more years hence? Voice your vision often. It may be idealistic but should seem possible. It should be simple, straightforward, and short. For example:

> "Our COPC program will decrease drug use by youth in the community in five years and will do this with the active participation of youth."

Step 5 - The mission: how will it be acted upon? While the vision comes mostly from the heart, the mission comes mostly from the brain. The group states its purpose, who the COPC team is, what it aims to achieve, and for whom. The team should re-evaluate its mission every year.

> "Our COPC program is a community-based team who, in cooperation with local medical providers and other health care professionals, is dedicated to improving the general health and environment of our community and doing this especially for and with our children so that they may grow without the influence of drugs."

Step 6 - The goals: what major actions lead to that vision and mission? Next, the COPC team should delineate realistic goals. They can be broken down into long and short range goals.

Goal One   Construct a youth activities center.

Goal Two   Establish drug education and counseling in all levels of the public schools.

Goal Three   Lobby for strong anti-drug laws locally and in the state.

Step 7 - The objectives: how can the goals be broken down into action steps? After consensus is achieved on the goals, outline objectives and corresponding activities as specifically as possible. For example:

Goal One   Construct a youth activities center.

> **Objective One** - Design the center
> > *Activity One* - Query youth as to what they want (who: Bob and Laurie; when: report back in two months; how: focus groups).
> > *Activity Two* - Look at other communities' centers (who: Jan; when: report back in two months; how: site visits to three established centers in adjacent counties).

> **Objective Two** - Raise funds
> > *Activity One* - Plan fundraising campaign (who: fundraising subcommittee; when: report back at next meeting)
> > *Activity Two* - Investigate public funds (who: Dorothy; when: report back with list in three months).

Step 8 - Strategies and activities. What are the specific tasks needed? Specify the means through which the objectives will be met. What specific actions and plans are needed to implement the intervention? Specify the number of expected participants, the measurements to be monitored, and the analyses to be performed.

Step 9 - Performance evaluation: are you making progress? Are the objectives being achieved? Failure to check progress repeatedly, in measurable terms, accounts for most of the failures in strategic planning.

Step 10 - Sustainability: can you keep it going? Revisit the strategic planning process often. Doing this renews the group, ensures that the mission is in step with the community, and often leads to recruitment of fresh membership.

CONSENSUS: THE PROCESS OF DECISION MAKING

A point echoed by many COPC practitioners is that establishing consensus within their teams for major decisions is one of the key ingredients of a successful process. Those given management authority by the team should unilaterally make day to day decisions on operational issues. Consensus on values, vision, mission, goals, and objectives facilitates decisive action by managers. Second guessing and reworking are minimized.

Taking votes prematurely usually leads to threatening divisions and disengagement by those who lose the vote. At times there may be one or two individuals who hold out against the group. Use persuasive data, patience, and attentiveness. An alienated individual will infect others with a negative point of view, and a hostile environment can result. Naysaying can seriously damage the prospects for success of COPC, especially since participation is typically voluntary. If a person cannot be convinced to go along with the other members, the facilitator should summarize that view, acknowledge it, value it, and point out that the overall group is committed to the directions it has adopted. This way, opportunities to engage dissenters productively in other parts of the group's work will be clearer. If consensus cannot be reached the group may decide that a certain percentage, i.e., two-thirds, of the total voting members is needed to pass any issue. If a vote or issue is divided equally, further study and clarification are called for prior to decision making. In fact, if an issue is controversial it will be better to hold off a vote until more informal discussion can occur.

Finally, leaders and managers need to be clear that a group decision has been accepted and will be acted on, even when it is different from an individual's own initial goals (see Figure. 4.1). If this doesn't occur, the COPC process will fail as the group members experience a loss of ownership. By enthusiastically and successfully assisting the implementation of a consensus decision, leaders gain legitimacy.

CONFLICT MANAGEMENT AND RESOLUTION

Don't take it personally. Resolve conflict by concentrating on the issues. Many leaders care deeply about their investment of time and effort. Thus, when a challenge comes, the tendency is to take it as a personal failing. People sometimes, therefore, become defensive or redirect attention from themselves by challenging the other individual. This emotional response

Figure 4.1: Gradients of Agreement

Group Facilitation Skills
Putting participatory values into practice

Gradients of Agreement

Endorsement	"I like it."
Endorsement with a minor point of contention	"Basically I like it."
Agreement with reservations	"I can live with it."
Abstain	"I have no opinion."
Stand aside	"I don't like this, but I don't want to hold up the group."
Formal disagreement, but willing to go with majority	"I want my disagreement noted in writing, but I'll support the decision."
Formal disagreement, with request to be absolved of responsibility for implementation	"I don't want to stop anyone else, but I don't want to be involved in implementing it."
Block	"I veto the proposal."

This is the Community at Work *Gradients of Agreement Scale*.
The scale makes it easier for participants to be honest. Using it, members can register less-than-wholehearted support without fearing that their statement will be interpreted as a veto.

Community at Work © 1998

is counterproductive and causes the group to polarize, and the real underlying problem becomes secondary.[12]

Avoid the tendency to personalize criticism or challenge the critic by making sure the team understands that problems, disagreements, and failures are a natural part of group maturation and productive action. Criticism may have validity, but it may have more to do with the COPC team's processes than with an individual. Success of the COPC process requires that the group progressively diffuse authority and responsibility, so that failures—like successes—can be shared as part of the team's work, rather than a reflection on a person's character.

Value the differences among people. Different people will have different ways of reaching goals. In these differences lie the strength of the group. There are often people in the group who, because of their congenial personalities or observational skills, become confidants of others. They can play the valuable leadership role of understanding and expressing underlying group dynamics that are not directly surfacing at meetings and key the group into problems and issues before they become disproportionately large or personalized. A COPC project in Lubec, Me, had an instructive way of formalizing this, as shown in Example 4.2.

There are five possible approaches to resolving conflict (see Table 4.2): *avoid* the conflict when its importance is low all the way around; *accommodate* when the issue's importance is low but the relationship with the other person is important; *compete* when there is little value to a future interpersonal relationship, the stakes are critical, and there are clearly only two opposing alternatives; *compromise* when a future relationship is important and an alternative approach is acceptable and workable; *collaborate* when both the relationship and the result are highly important and seek alternative means to agreement. Each of these strategies has its appropriate place, but collaboration is usually desired because both parties obtain their immediate goals and retain, or strengthen, their relationship as well. Collaboration begets "win/win" situations. It requires time, patience, and effort.

Get to a win/win situation by using a problem solving approach (see Table 4.3). When it's clear that an impasse has been reached, go back to the mission, vision, and values of the group. Take the problem apart and redefine it, if possible, in the context of the COPC team's goals and objectives, the causes of the conflict, and options for solution. Depersonalize it, and eliminate individual positions. Discuss the problem, its sources, and potential solutions in the context of the conflicting individuals' basic goals; they often turn out to be the same. The differences are more often in style and process. Arrive at a solution by group consensus. This is often easily accomplished by brainstorming, subsequent discussion, and then a nomi-

---

EXAMPLE 4.2
Maintenance Crews

A Team Actively Manages Group Process
Lubec, Maine
Author: Ben Thompson

There are times in the life of any group when boredom, frustration, or anger sets in. To prevent these feelings from putting the team on a downward spiral, our group had a "maintenance crew," two people who attended to the group's dynamics, the emotional tension, and the energy level. When they sensed boredom or frustration, they got the group up out of their chairs for a short break or to do what we called "energizers," anything that gets the heart pumping and the mind unglued from the problem at hand for two to three minutes such as jumping jacks, a yoga exercise, or musical chairs. Our group also liked trust building activities. One was to lift a person off the floor and over everyone's head. As our group became more comfortable, we learned to express our feelings on issues. We actually performed spectrograms in which we physically arranged ourselves in a line representing the spectrum of our positions on an issue with those feeling strongly in one direction on one end and those feeling the other way at the opposite end.

---

nal group technique (see Chapter 5). Finally, encourage those who still have an issue with the proposed solution to voice their perspective. This will usually lead to a final consensus, which may need slight tinkering, and an investment in it by all parties.

NEGOTIATION

The Harvard Negotiation Project offers similar advice on negotiating through problems.[13] Fruitful negotiation can be summarized in four basic points. One, attend to the people involved in the dispute only enough to separate them from the problem. Two, focus on the people's interests, not their positions. Three, generate a variety of possibilities for addressing in-

TABLE 4.2
Strategies for Conflict Resolution

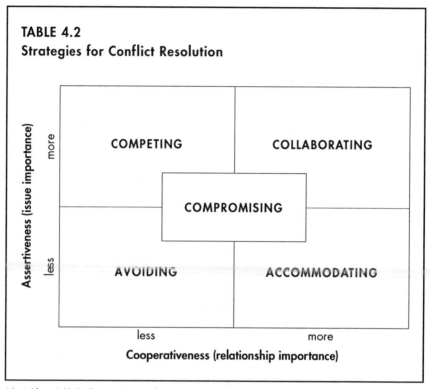

Adapted from: Ruble TL, Thomas K. Support for a two dimensional model of conflict behavior. *Organizational Behavior and Human Performance.* June 1976; 16:143-55.

terests before attempting to decide what to do. Invent options for mutual gain by consulting the views of different experts, and invent possible agreements that speak only to partial solutions (a whole solution may be hiding therein). Four, insist that the criteria for evaluating the possible solutions be objective. Examples include market value, precedent, scientific judgment, professional standards, efficiency, costs, what a court would decide, specific and published moral standards, equality, tradition, and reciprocity.

The Harvard research on negotiations also produced four pieces of advice about how to communicate during problem resolution. One, listen actively and acknowledge what the other has said. Hear not only what comes out of the other person's mouth, but also what seems to be meant. Phrases like "I hear you saying that..." can be helpful ways to hypothesize about and test whether you are hearing what the other is saying. Two,

---

TABLE 4.3
Problem Solving Steps

1. Review group mission, vision, and values.

2. Redefine problem in context of goals and objectives, and potential solutions.

3. Eliminate personal positions.

4. Discuss problem at the level of individual basic goals.

5. Solve problem by group consensus techniques.

---

speak to be understood. Talk to the other person in a way that reflects your understanding of how the other understands you and the world. This may sometimes be assisted through the use of private and confidential channels. It is often helpful to limit the number of parties involved in a dispute. Three, while trying to hear what the other person means, talk only about yourself, not about them. Say, "I feel let down," instead of "you let me down." Four, speak for a purpose. Avoid offering new or significant statements about the problem or preferred options until you know what you want the other person to hear or what you want to learn. Know what you are about to say well enough to know why it is the right thing for the other person to hear or for you to learn.

MEETINGS, MEETINGS, MEETINGS ! ! !

While meetings can be fun, unless they are run properly they can also be an immense waste of time, boring, and non-productive. It is critical to the COPC process to run crisp and effective meetings. The following key points can help[14]:

1. Prepare for the meeting.

Have a clear agenda of items to be covered and decisions to be made. Send the agenda out ahead of time so team members can think about it. At the beginning of the meeting, ask if there are items to be added. A clear agenda at the beginning of the meeting will allow the facilitator to keep an eye on the clock and ensure that each item is covered. Cover each item; forgetting an item might offend the person who put it on the agenda. If there is not enough time to cover the entire agenda, prioritize and cover the most important or largest issues first. Items can be postponed explicitly until the next meeting but they should never be merely dropped or forgotten.

2. Add a social dimension.

Occasionally include social activities. These bind people together and help create commitment to the group. One suggestion is to have refreshments or food available before the meeting. This helps people start talking so they will be "warmed up" at the beginning of the meeting. Other suggestions include periodic potlucks or outings to celebrate a success or holiday. Keep to a strict timetable and do not let the social part of the meeting dominate.

3. Facilitate—don't direct!

Each COPC team member has a chance to exercise leadership by helping facilitate interaction in the group. A good facilitator draws out ideas and opinions from as many members as possible, attaches a valuing comment to them, and adds a directing question designed to elicit an answer that keeps the group on the agenda item. A good facilitator learns to endure long periods of silence (up to 10 or 20 seconds) after posing a question for discussion. Most people will say something before that time has elapsed, and a discussion will be underway. When the discussion strays from the point, the facilitator must make the decision to let it go on because it is productive or to bring the group back to the agenda item at hand. If the discussion is allowed to stray, the facilitator should keep track of the time and eventually refocus the group on the agenda item.

4. Always identify the next step.

Another key to facilitation is to bring agenda items to closure. Summarize the discussion, offer a concrete action step, and achieve consensus. If an item is tabled, identify a new discussion date. Closure provides a sense of accomplishment and a sense of where the group is going.

5. Be on time!

This applies to starting the meeting and, especially, to ending the meeting. It lends credibility to the group's management ability and ensures promptness at future meetings. Place unfinished items on the next agenda rather than drag on and have people trickle out of the meeting. If your team members know that meetings start and finish on time, they are more likely to attend because they can plan their time more reliably.

6. Put it in writing.

A written record of a meeting, or minutes, saves a lot of confusion later on, and it provides information for members who could not attend. To be readable and useful the minutes should be concise (1-2 pages maximum), in outline form by agenda item, and should focus primarily on decisions made and timetables for activities to be performed. It is not necessary to recreate the meeting by putting too much detail in the minutes or by quoting individuals' input.

7. Difficult people.

Clearly a meeting with a group of diverse people can be expected to take on its own personality. But several types of persons can be notably problematic:

a. Those who tend to dominate.

b. Those who never say anything.

c. Those who must be continually educated about the expected outcome and process because they have other agendas.

d. Those who block the discussion with negativity or other means.

A facilitator who appreciates these problems can use specific techniques to remedy them.

Some participants seem to dominate meetings. They may have a position of bureaucratic authority that leads them to believe that all the other team members need to hear their opinions. Or they may be so enthusiastic that they don't realize they are dominating. Domination can be particularly troublesome when they either have a negative attitude ("that's been tried before and failed") or for some reason are out to directly challenge the group's directions.

The best way to deal with this is not to take them on directly, but to defuse them and make them allies through recognizing their personal contribution ("Thank you, Bob, for your observation. What is your point of view on this particular topic, Louise?"). Soliciting input from other team members is a good tactic. The use of the nominal group technique outlined in Chapter 5 is particularly effective because it systematically asks all participants for their input. Another method is to draw difficult individuals aside after a meeting and listen to their concerns privately.

COPC AS AN APPROACH TO SUCCESS
IN A MANAGED CARE WORLD

The importance of managed care continues to grow. According to the 1996 *HMO-PPO Digest*,[15] over 67 million Americans were enrolled in HMOs in 1995 (see Figure 4.2). Enrollment in HMOs more than doubled between 1988 and 1995 and increased by 23 percent in 1995 alone. Forty-five percent of contracts with ancillary providers were capitated in 1995, as were 45 percent of contracts with specialists. Thirty-five percent of contracts with hospitals used capitation.

Whether it has yet become prominent in your community, the growth of managed care signals more than capitation; it signals recognition that the US has at least 20 percent more doctors and hospital beds than it requires. It signals a shift in the health sector from a regulatory model to a market model. It reflects payors' insistence that the value of health services must be proven. The pressures are not going away soon. Our population is aging, with people in the mammoth "baby boom" demographic bulge about to enter their chronic care years. And, health care spending that continues growing faster than inflation cannot go on indefinitely.

If you envision a growth strategy for your organization, a proactive shift toward COPC can prepare you and your health care provider colleagues for aggressive, effective, and socially responsible participation in managed care.[16] Efficient management of the well-being of an enrolled population is the care provider's imperative under managed care.

Managed care requires a health plan, and it requires caregivers to broaden their focus from the needs of the individual patient to the health of the population they serve. COPC represents a set of activities through which a primary care practice attempts to bridge the traditional gap between individual and community health. Thus, managed care and COPC

FIGURE 4.2: Managed Care's Impact So Far: Enrollment in HMOs

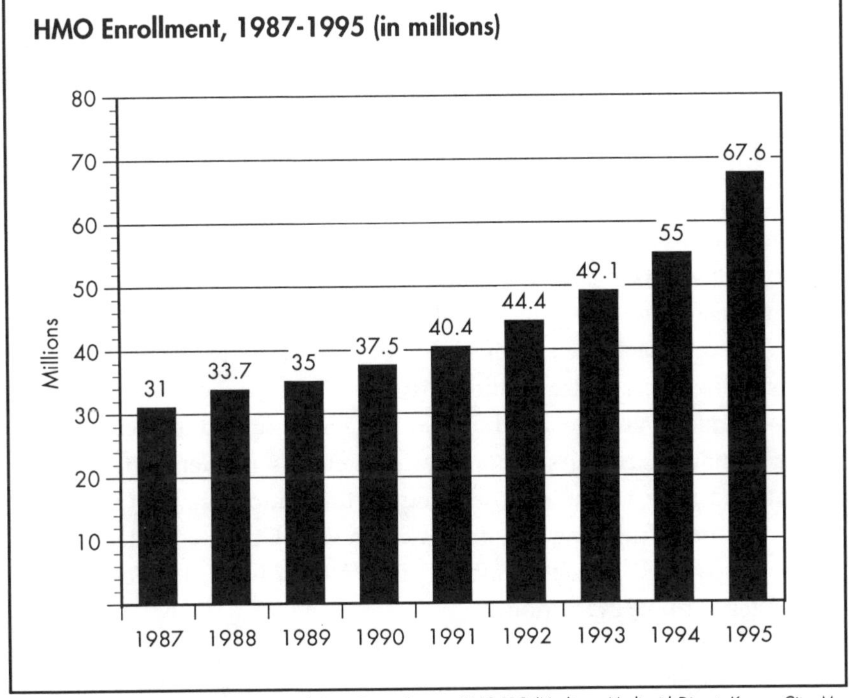

HMO Enrollment, 1987-1995 (in millions)

Sources: Hoechst Marion Roussel Managed Care Digest Series, *HMO-PPO/Medicare-Medicaid Digest*. Kansas City, Mo: Hoechst Marion Roussel; 1997. Health Care Financing Administration.

share a need to provide suitable care to an individual patient while endeavoring to improve the overall health status of the communities they serve. Managed care and COPC use some of the same techniques: identification, intervention, and evaluation.

There are several key differences, however.[17] A managed care plan is usually focused on financial health and performance while a COPC process more often arises out of a sense of civic duty and health concerns. Managed care companies will often have more resources than a COPC team to invest in a community project, but may choose not to do so because of competitive or profit concerns. Example 4.3 illustrates potential intersections between managed care and COPC.

As payment for health services shifts from fee-for-service to capitation, it becomes increasingly appealing for managed care companies and other provider organizations to invest in strategies to keep their covered

---

EXAMPLE 4.3
COPC and Managed Care

Managed Care Companies Can Be Partners, Too
Authors: Richard Roberts and Richard Bogue

A managed care company with a Medicare risk contract establishes a senior outreach safety program in coordination with a local COPC team that wants to address the same problem. The company's catchment area overlaps with the COPC community and is divided into four regions, each the responsibility of a nurse coordinator paid by the managed care organization (MCO). The residence of every insured person over age 65 who lives alone is identified on a computerized map. Each nurse coordinator visits the residence of every identified senior to assess the safety of the senior's home (e.g., removing throw rugs, installing safety bars, etc.). COPC volunteers are then dispatched to each senior's home with a written checklist of changes to make in the home.

The $500,000 investment (computer software, nurses' salaries, safety equipment) yields $2 million a year in savings for the entire population by reducing the incidence of hip fractures and other injuries. The MCO's savings are proportional to the number of affected seniors who were MCO enrollees. For example, if half are MCO enrollees, this would result in a $1,000,000 savings for the MCO.

This is an example of a managed care company doing well by doing good and by partnering with a COPC team. The favorable short-term financial implications give companies an incentive to institute such a program. As part of the COPC team, the managed care company reaps social marketing benefits and lowers its direct project costs because the partnership gets help from community volunteers for some program activities.

---

populations healthy, which can be much less expensive than paying for their illnesses. In fact, an increasing number of providers are considering whether to assume the financial risk of health care and whether they might produce better outcomes for their customers and themselves.[16] Whether by managed care organizations or provider-sponsored health plans, these strategies encourage plans to reach out to their members, outside of the clinical setting, and involve a wide array of professionals and community members in intervention objectives. In this way, the goals of managed care and COPC are congruent. Managed care can offer the financial incentives and resources needed to address community health objectives; COPC can provide the specific techniques (see Example 4.4).

LEGAL ISSUES

Legal issues seem to complicate many American lives. Fortunately, this is most uncommon for COPC. A fundamental legal question for a COPC team is the organizational structure it will adopt. Most projects will be seen in the eyes of the law as a subset of the COPC sponsors (primary care practice, public health department, hospital, school board, etc.) or as an ill-defined community activity. Some COPC efforts, especially as they become larger, more complex, and expensive, may want to consider a more formal structure. Incorporation as a non-profit, tax exempt organization (i.e., a 501(c)(3) organization) may confer certain advantages by providing structure, legal continuity, tax incentives for fundraising, and tax reductions. Some community partnerships, however, worry that incorporation will lead away from the ideals of consensus, equal participation, and inclusiveness, and toward bureaucratization.

Another legal issue to consider is antitrust. There may be instances where a health care concern (e.g., practice, hospital, or other business) may feel disadvantaged by a competitor's use of COPC activities and allege restraint of trade or other unfair business practices. An example would be two competitors (e.g., two independent medical groups) who collaborate on a COPC intervention and (intentionally or not) increase their share of the local health care market, to the detriment of a third group. This risk can be minimized by having wide community involvement in the project and by having the broadly representative COPC team, or the community advisory committee, rather than the competitors, decide on and sponsor the intervention.

A final legal consideration is a claim against the COPC project for damages resulting from the project (e.g., an individual injured due to negligent blood drawing, a slip and fall at a COPC event, an aggrieved com-

---

EXAMPLE 4.4

COPC Within Managed Care
A Pregnant Idea
Authors: Richard Bogue and Richard Roberts

The Solano Partnership Health Plan (SPH) north of the San Francisco Bay Area operates the Growing Together Perinatal Program (GTPP). SPH identifies members who are pregnant, and a perinatal case manager conducts a risk assessment over the phone. For those at low risk, GTPP provides prenatal care, educational materials, referrals, and transportation to support services, interpreter services, counseling, and ombudsman services. Of the 618 pregnant women enrolled in the first year, 15 percent were high risk and qualified for specialized services including special education, monthly contacts by the case manager, compliance monitoring, and priority referrals.

Comparing birth outcomes for one year (1996-97), gestational age for case managed neonatal intensive care unit (NICU) babies was 2.25 weeks greater than for non-case managed NICU babies. Case managed babies also had average birth weights 370 grams higher than non-case managed babies.

At an annual cost of $108,635, costs per member were $175.78. Using baseline NICU utilization and per diem rates for these patients, had GTPP not been in place, an additional $99,005 might have been spent. These savings suggest a return on investment of 91 percent. Any provider showing savings of that magnitude makes itself a very attractive contractor for health care services as well as a place known for quality.

---

petitor). Insurance to protect against such claims is usually provided through the general and professional liability policies of the COPC sponsoring organization(s). It is important to determine the extent of coverage for COPC activities under such policies. It may also be wise to protect the leaders of the COPC project with a "directors and officers" liability policy, depending on the structure and activities of the project. Increasingly, larger provider organizations, like hospitals, are not only well insured against liability resulting from the efforts of their volunteers, but also provide health insurance for them.

The more complex and ambitious a COPC project becomes, the more it may want to consider obtaining expert legal advice. In the law, as in health care, "an ounce of prevention is worth a pound of cure and can avoid a ton of trouble."

REFERENCES

1. Weber M. *The Theory of Social and Economic Organizations*. Henderson AM, Parsons T, trans-ed. New York, NY: Oxford University Press;1947.
2. Gardner JW. *On Leadership*. New York, NY: Free Press; 1990.
3. Pollard CW. Epilogue. In: Bogue R, Hall CH, eds. *Health Network Innovations*. Chicago, Ill: American Hospital Publishing Inc; 1997;405-410.
4. Goodspeed SW. *Community Stewardship: Applying the Five Principles of Contemporary Governance*. Chicago, Ill: AHA Press; 1997.
5. Drucker PF. *Managing the Nonprofit Organization: Principles and Practice*. New York, NY: Harper Collins Publishers; 1990.
6. Dunham RB. *Organizational Behavior: People and Process in Management*. Homewood, Ill: 1984.
7. Filley AC. *The Complete Manager: What Works and What Doesn't*. Middleton, Wis: Greenbriar Press; 1978.
8. *The Community Collaboration Manual*. Washington, DC: National Assembly of Voluntary Health and Social Organizations. 1991.
9. Amundson B, Elder W. *A Prelude to Strategic Planning: Making Your Organization and Community Fit for Success*. Chicago, Ill: Hospital Research and Educational Trust; 1989.
10. American Hospital Association Staff. *The Strategic Planning Workbook*. Chicago, Ill: Hospital Research and Educational Trust; 1989.
11. Bogue RJ, Hall CH, eds. *Health Network Innovations*. Chicago, Ill: AHA Press; 1997.
12. Ruble TL, Thomas K. Support for a two dimensional model of conflict behavior. *Organizational Behavior and Human Performance*. June 1976;16:143-55.
13. Fisher R, Ury W. *Getting to Yes: Negotiating Agreement Without Giving In*. 2nd ed. Boston, Mass: Penguin Books; 1991.
14. Zander A. *Making Groups Effective*. San Francisco, Calif: Jossey-Bass Publishers, Inc; 1982.
15. *Managed Care Digest Series: HMO-PPO Digest*. Kansas City, Mo: Hoechst Marion Roussel; 1996.
16. *Rural Managed Care: Patterns & Prospects*. Minneapolis, Minn: University of Minnesota, Rural Health Research Center; 1997.
17. Pyenson BS, ed. *Calculated Risk: A Provider's Guide to Assessing and Controlling the Financial Risk of Managed Care*. Chicago, Ill: AHA Press; 1995.
18. Rohrer JE. *Planning for Community-Oriented Health Systems*. Washington, DC: APHA; 1996.

CHAPTER 5

Techniques for Developing a Community Partnership

Nina Wallerstein

Barbara Sheline

ABSTRACT

Community participation is critical to the success of the COPC process. To ensure a collaborative effort with the community, the COPC team should perform the following five tasks: (1) As individuals, assess their own resources and interest in becoming partners with the community, including all of its cultural, ethnic, and social backgrounds. (2) Engage the community from the start by identifying relevant social networks and leaders, then create structures for participation, such as the community advisory board and volunteer opportunities, initiate a community visioning process, and gather data on community perceptions, needs, and resources. (3) Identify and set priorities among health problems using consensus-building techniques. (4) Enlist the community for the intervention, setting goals, devising strategies, determining resources and potential barriers, and establishing a time line. (5) Evaluate outcomes, sharing this responsibility with the community. COPC teams have a variety of consensus-building techniques at their disposal, including brainstorming, modified Delbecq or nominal group technique, Delphi prioritization, problem analysis, action planning, visioning, force-field analysis, social analysis, focus groups, and group facilitation.

INTRODUCTION

Earlier writings about COPC viewed "community" primarily as a target population. This target population, defined often as a geographic region or subpopulation with a defined health problem, would receive needs assessments and interventions from the provider team. As indicated in Chapter 1, this book argues that COPC has matured and is now a process in which community participation is a core element in success. Many techniques for achieving participation are described in this chapter; not all will be used by everyone practicing COPC. COPC teams will need to manage their priorities carefully and make selective use of the suggested methods.

WHY THE COMMUNITY SHOULD BE A PARTNER IN COPC

Community participation has underpinned much of primary care in the US since the 1960s, when federally funded health centers first were required to establish "maximum feasible participation" by citizen boards. In the last decade and a half, with the surge of community coalitions[1] and community organizing in the health arena,[2,3] partnerships and other collaborative efforts have emerged, and community capacity has increased. The movement for healthy cities and communities throughout the US, initiated by the World Health Organization and supported by organizations such as the National Civic League and the Health Care Forum, has strengthened the collaborative philosophy. Local governments are mobilizing communities, collaborating with other sectors, and reducing social inequities.[4] Community leadership is now crucial to improving quality of life at the local level.

With the advent of managed care, health care systems are seeking to stay within fixed or shrinking budgets. By working with the community, they can identify perceived needs and use existing community resources, thus avoiding duplication and promoting systems that have proven their success. In other words, they can avoid reinventing the wheel.

Community participation offers innumerable benefits to COPC. It ensures that the process represents the perceptions, needs, culture, beliefs, and priorities of the community. On the other hand, interventions based on health providers' priorities or health statistics alone may fail because they have little to do with the community's felt needs or motivation to act.[5] Community members can help to identify needed services as well as community resources relevant to the selection of strategies. McKnight's idea of "community regeneration" reminds us that community members need opportunities to bring their "gifts" to the table.[6] Most important, community partnership can ensure community ownership and motivation

---

EXAMPLE 5.1
Defining Community

A Community Meeting Defines the Community
Seminary, Mississippi
Author: Barbara Sheline

A community health center in rural Seminary, Miss, defined its community as the southern end of the county and used radio, television, and newspapers to advertise a community meeting on local health problems. But people came from northern parts of the county as well, changing the staff's definition of community. Over the next three years, the health center worked with residents countywide. An advisory board was formed, and the board ultimately identified lonely elders as the subpopulation around whom to design an intervention.

---

and can increase members' capacity to assume responsibility for their community's health and well-being.

Community empowerment is both a process and an outcome. It is a means to gain control over the conditions affecting one's personal and community life. People remain powerless when acted upon as "objects," or informed what programs will work best for them. To become empowered, they must help make the choices.[7,8,9] An empowered community is better able to solve problems, bring in needed resources, and tap into existing strengths. Enhanced psychological and community empowerment itself, with its greater sense of community responsibility, leads to improved health regardless of the COPC intervention[10,11] (see Example 5.1).

DEFINING THE COMMUNITY

Your first question may be, "So, what is my community... a neighborhood, a town, my patients, the senior citizens in my county?" The answers often depend on the type of participation you want to engage. During the COPC process, the community may define itself. Your success will depend on your flexibility to work with the community that wants to join you (see Example 5.1).

A community is a group of people with something in common, e.g., a language, geographical boundaries, age, attendance at a primary care clinic, shared cause, bond of identity, history or values. They perceive a commonality among themselves.[12] They can include groups drawn together by mutual interest, ethnicity, disease experience, or organizational affiliation, such as environmental or African-American organizations, gay and lesbian activists, church members, university students, or employees in a worksite. A sense of community among people can motivate them to improve health conditions among their members.

CHALLENGES AND REWARDS

Those who have worked with communities to bring about change will "recognize the enormous journey, the Himalayan trek, from idea to action, from expressed value to concrete results."[13] The process is fluid, dynamic, at times fast-paced and at times slow, and always requires long-term commitment. The old axiom "plan and then implement the plan" is too simplistic. To succeed, community plans must be open to permutations and reformulations as the process unfolds. Unexpected obstacles can surface, such as staff turnover or a change in local leadership. Partnership means spending the time to develop trust, so that unexpected directions or setbacks can be seen as part of a long-term process that will continue.

Although community participation has been increasingly recognized as important, most health professionals are not trained in community organizing or involvement. Motivated practitioners are still often assumed to be more important than community participation.[14] While COPC teams have historically solicited community response to the ideas proposed by health professionals, we propose that health professionals and community leaders work collaboratively. Community leaders can mentor health professionals on how to engage their communities. Collaboration can result in many possible levels of community participation,[15] as shown in Figure 5.1.

FIVE TASKS OF COMMUNITY PARTICIPATION

If you are beginning the process of working collaboratively on a health problem, use the five tasks presented below as a strategy. We propose that

FIGURE 5.1: Community Participation Continuum

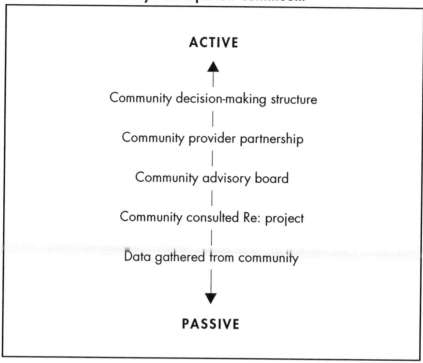

you start with task one, but the others are not necessarily meant to be performed sequentially.

1. **Assess** your own resources as a health professional and your interest in becoming partners with the community.

2. **Engage** the community by identifying the relevant social networks and leaders.

3. **Prioritize** health problems using consensus-building techniques.

4. **Develop** strategies to enlist community involvement in the intervention.

5. **Evaluate** outcomes, involving the community from the start.

In the sections below, we discuss group facilitation skills to accomplish each task.

Methods for Task One: Health Professional Self-Assessment

Before beginning work, the project initiation team discussed in Chapter 3 would benefit from an internal assessment of their attitudes, resources, cultural sensitivities, and capabilities for fostering community participation. The team might conduct a brainstorming session (see specifics later on in this chapter), asking four questions:[16]

1. "What are the **strengths** of our project initiation team and health facility for working with the community?"

2. "What are our **weaknesses**, as individuals and as an institution?"

3. "What **benefits** do we stand to gain?"

4. "What **dangers** do we face?" (For example, we may have to share control.)

An assessment of cultural sensitivities can help staff understand their abilities to work with people from different cultural, ethnic, and social backgrounds (see Appendix 5.1 for the Berkeley survey about attitudes towards patients from different backgrounds, which can be adapted to more general questions). Many health professionals are of a different race, ethnicity, economic, or educational background than the community with whom they desire to work. They may lack the cultural competencies to work in communities of color, and they may not appreciate the unique characteristics of these communities, such as the style of their social networks.[17] Health professionals must be careful not to see themselves as "empowering others" as much as giving up power so that the community has an opportunity to develop its own.[18]

Self-assessment must address people's values and willingness, their skills and resources to engage in collaborative work. After this self-assessment, the project initiation team should make a decision on their model of participation and whether the benefits outweigh the extra commitment of time and resources when working with a community. Once this decision is made, then the team will be able to better strategize how to confront the barriers they are likely to encounter within themselves and the community.

Any collaboration among community members, especially if they represent different cultural or ethnic groups, eventually leads to a need for conflict resolution. Much has been written about the conflicts that come from differences in needs and assumptions: from professionals, who are often driven by scientific data, and from community members, who may be driven by high profile issues.[19-21] Hold regular meetings between the COPC team and community representatives to discuss assumptions (facilitation methods are presented later). Potential conflicts can turn into opportunities for strengthening trust in the community process.

Methods for Task Two: Engaging the Community

Follow these four steps to enter a community in a respectful manner:

1. Learn to listen. Listening for community issues requires skill, patience, and an attitude of openness and discovery, the same as when you establish rapport with patients. It takes time to uncover the many undercurrents of opinions, politics, history, social networks, and values that may divide or connect members of a community. You should recognize that there are things you may never learn about the community, but this should not doom your efforts as long as your approach is respectful.[22] In the early stages, ask two questions: "Who are the leaders to talk with?" and "What do we want to learn from them?" Disclose your intentions openly, smile, make eye contact, and communicate your interest in building a relationship. A third party who knows you can facilitate your entry into the community. Ask leaders about how they perceive the issues confronting the community and the community's abilities to confront them (see Example 5.2).

2. Create structures for community participation. Create structure by forming a community advisory board and soliciting volunteers. Do this by working with two types of civic leadership:

▶ Formal leadership, such as the mayor, city council, chamber of commerce, school principals, church ministers, hospital chief executive officers, service organization presidents, or heads of networks of social service providers.

EXAMPLE 5.2
Listening to the Community

Health Center Learns to Draw in Latino Population
Codman Square Community Health Center, Boston, Massachusetts
Author: Suzanne Cashman

The Codman Square Community Health Center was incorporated in 1975 by community activists seeking to revitalize an urban community and fill a vacuum left by the disappearance of local private physicians. The center sought from the beginning to foster community empowerment. Staff were encouraged to develop formal and informal relationships with other community groups and services. But despite connections with the community, the staff and board members were aware that they lacked the capacity to look at the epidemiology of community health issues, and that health programs had been developed and administered with community members noticeably absent. Staff were selected for COPC training through a local hospital's preventive medicine residency/fellowship program, supported by the Kellogg Foundation and the Health Resources and Services Administration.

Continued on the following page.

▶ Informal leaders, such as representatives of neighborhood associations, consumer advocacy groups, or mutual aid societies, or just well-known people in a church congregation or neighborhood. Ask the question, "To whom do people turn for advice or assistance?" If any names are mentioned several times, it is likely that these people are informal leaders who might be willing to help.

Within these two groups, look for a skilled community organizer who can mentor the health professionals. Look for potential members of the community advisory board or for consultants. Some leaders may have the power to block COPC efforts if they feel threatened or ignored; identify them and determine how best to work with them.

Continued from the previous page.

One of the clinicians eager to learn the COPC approach was a nurse practitioner who was fluent in Spanish. She was aware that, while Latinos made up about 13 percent of the health center's denominator community, only 4% of Codman Square's patients had Latino surnames.

She asked her patients and other Latino members of the community what they viewed as their major health problems and learned that it was the health center itself. Many viewed the center as unwelcoming because few staff spoke Spanish, signs were in English only, and staff were not particularly culturally competent.

Working with members of the Latino community, the nurse practitioner developed a series of free health promotion/disease prevention modules in Spanish and conducted a 12-session semi nar series for staff in cultural competency and diversity appreciation. Mini-health fairs were held as part of an outreach effort to the Latino community. In addition, the health center hired a bilingual receptionist and modified its signs and taped telephone messages so that they were in Spanish as well as English. A year and a half later, the percentage of health center patients with Latino surnames had risen to 25%.

Ask leaders to invite the project initiation team to meetings to explain the COPC process and gain support. Then issue personal invitations to attend a community advisory board organizing meeting to individuals whom you want as members.

(See Chapter 4 for more information on how to develop partnerships with community leaders and organizations, and Chapter 3 on the use of community advisory boards).

Besides the community advisory board, develop a cadre of volunteers. The word volunteer has typically meant middle class women and retired people. Today, however, over 47% of Americans 18 or over serve in unpaid positions. Therefore, the pool of potential volunteers may be sizeable in even the smallest communities. Your volunteers might be called community health workers, peer educators, community health representatives, health *promotoras*, or lay health workers. The community health worker is a member of the community who may have leadership characteristics or merely a strong desire to improve the community's health and well-being.

Increasingly in the developing world and the United States, community health workers serve as outreach workers who extend health interventions into their social networks and reach otherwise difficult-to-reach populations, such as migrant farmworkers, communities with low prenatal care or hard-to-identify diabetics, tuberculosis patients on long-term medication, or teen populations who would prefer to talk with peers.[23] Some programs pay community health workers, others do not (see Example 5.3).

The following guidelines will help you succeed in recruiting and managing volunteers and community health workers:

▶ Recruit them as you would staff members, with job descriptions clearly outlined.

▶ Interview them to assess their interest and the level of commitment they are willing to make.

▶ Train for specific tasks, e.g., administering a questionnaire. Some community leaders or other volunteers may be qualified to be trainers.

▶ Provide ongoing support through scheduled training, evaluation, and rewards such as certificates, thank-you letters, award ceremonies, or through more tangible benefits such as discounts on services.

▶ Provide early and frequent opportunities for success, such as an easily administered questionnaire.

▶ Encourage the development of group cohesiveness and broader purpose through regularly scheduled meetings.

▶ Start from a partnership model to involve the volunteers in decision-making from the outset.

▶ Eventually allow volunteers or community health workers to take on their own projects.

EXAMPLE 5.3
Community Health Workers/Volunteers

A COPC Process Includes Community Members
Franklin, West Virginia
Author: David Cockley

Pendleton Community Care (PCC) in West Virginia identified the need for key community listeners to articulate the needs of the community and provide a short feedback loop for determining how community interventions were perceived by the community's informal social network. PCC also saw the need for health promoters to disseminate health promotion and disease prevention information.

To recruit key community listeners, PCC asked people in the community to identify others "who know about health issues." Thirty-five key community listeners were identified through a survey and through clinic patients and project supporters. Although PCC envisioned a formal structure in which the community listeners would meet regularly and provide formal feedback, the community listeners did not wish to assume this role. Most were willing to be an informal resource and provide feedback on specific interventions when asked individually.

After the subpopulations (elders, worksites, and teens) were chosen for the interventions, PCC wanted to identify key listeners and promoters within each network. With the teenagers, PCC utilized a network of informal health promoters within the high school. Each fall, a survey was administered to grades 9 - 12 asking teenagers to identify who among their peers they would go to for "counsel, advice and support." The top candidates were invited to become natural helpers. Following training on listening and referral skills, the natural helpers were provided with information on teen health issues. They then were able to refer students to needed services and help disseminate health information.

3. Create a community visioning process. The National Civic League's healthy community program and World Health Organization (WHO) Healthy Cities model suggest starting with a visioning activity to motivate people to become engaged in community change. Visioning may be done with different groups in the community, as part of town hall meetings, or as part of the COPC community board's early development. The idea of visioning is to let your imagination create a new world, without constraints, that you would want to live in five or 10 years from now. Here is one visioning scenario; others are presented later on.

> Ask each person to imagine he or she is floating above the community in a hot air balloon five years from now. Have everyone describe in writing what they see, in detail. Tell them to embrace possibilities, to refrain from thinking about costs, but instead to "dream as high as you can and imagine you have no obstacles."

4. Gather community data on perceptions, needs, and resources. Gathering information on community needs may be an early task of a newly formed community board, or it may be the COPC team's first step. COPC publicity events can facilitate data gathering, which in turn provides an opportunity to uncover potential members of the advisory board or COPC team. Here are five techniques:

A. Community social environment map and windshield survey
A social environment map includes the physical layout of the community; its resources; community leaders and organizations; social groupings, support networks, and communities that people identify with; level of community membership and belonging; social, political, or cultural constraints which detract from problem-solving; and history of problem resolution.[24]

Begin with your observations.[25] Even if you have lived in a community for a long time, take a fresh look. Perform a windshield survey; drive through neighborhoods and observe resources and places for meetings, such as restaurants, churches, laundromats, clubs, agencies. Observe conditions of homes, parks, and vehicles; activity level; and neighborliness. Stop and ask people to describe their community. Does it have a name or special characteristics? What is its history? Ask to whom people go for advice. Identify key social networks, such as neighborhood associations, recreation programs, adult education offerings, or senior centers. You may need to check the library or city hall records for this information.

B. Interviews

Talk to a cross-section of individuals to get their views on the priority health problems, informal networks, alternative systems of care, and anything else you or they might think is important to the COPC process. In addition to leaders, such as elementary school principals or church leaders, try to find some "known gripers" who may have different insights. Their opinions will be important when you are considering obstacles and barriers to your COPC project. Use individual interviews to share your ideas and goals.

Interview formats can range from informal and unstructured to very structured using a written questionnaire. The former tends to encourage a dialogue and open-ended discussion. On the other hand, the structured written interview will cover all the questions you have written down, but the answers may not reflect the subject's true feelings. It may be helpful to conduct your interviews somewhere in-between. For example, ask, "What are the priority health problems in this community that you think could or should be addressed?" This allows a spontaneous response, as opposed to a more closed-ended question such as, "Rank the following ten health problems from 1 to 10." More structured questions are best used after a series of open-ended interviews have identified the 10 or 15 problems mentioned most often.

C. Surveys

Develop a questionnaire. Volunteers or community health workers can help design and gather data through surveys. Their participation can also develop needed contacts with community support networks. Data may be more objective if volunteers gather data from groups to which they don't belong. In this way, their knowledge about different views in the community is also broadened.

Carefully designed questionnaires can produce a wealth of information (see Chapter 6 for techniques). Guidelines from the point of view of community implementation include[26]:

1. Identify categories of information to cover. Although COPC focuses on addressing health problems, a general first question about the core problems faced by the community will often elicit more information and also put people at ease. Some people may have a narrow view of health, considering only disease entities such as arthritis or hypertension. Questions strictly on health problems may inhibit people from thinking about problems such as adolescent pregnancy or violence. Include questions about social networks, community identity, history, strengths, and weaknesses.

2. Write a brief introduction to the COPC project with an assurance of confidentiality.

3. Develop questions about each category identified in the first step. Ensure the language is appropriate for ethnic, racial, or regional considerations. Develop neutral questions without bias and avoid double-barrelled questions that ask two questions simultaneously. Begin with easy-to-answer non-threatening questions and develop probes for in-depth responses to a few questions, rather than being satisfied with superficial answers.

4. Include a final question about subjects' interest in COPC and their willingness to volunteer.

5. Develop a cover form to record time, place, date, a common checklist of information such as type of organization or agency affiliation, and any other relevant information.

6. If your resources are limited, select and train a few interviewers to administer the questionnaire. They should understand the COPC process so they can garner support.

7. Look for existing validated instruments to which you can add questions. There is no need to reinvent a questionnaire if an existing form fits your needs.

8. Pilot test your questionnaire.

Conduct a survey. Community perceptions of issues and needs can be collected by sampling a representative cross-section of the community. You can distribute questionnaires at a convenient location (for example, a health fair or shopping mall), or you can use strict statistical sampling techniques. Surveys can serve multiple purposes: to collect specific data, to publicize the project, and to collect names of potential volunteers.

D. Focus groups and small group meetings
A focus group interview is a method to gain information from a small group, using a structured set of questions and allowing open-ended responses. Focus groups bring together community representatives from similar backgrounds to discuss community health issues, resources, and barriers to care. The results can suggest questions for formal surveys. They can also be used to pilot test a questionnaire. They may also strengthen existing networks and contribute to a health provider's base of support. The key to success is to be impartial and allow the focus group members to feel safe sharing ideas. The specific technique of conducting focus groups is described at the end of this chapter. A more thorough discussion of focus groups is provided in Chapter 8.

Methods for Task Three: Community Problem Prioritization
Small group consensus-building methods of problem prioritization and analysis enable health providers, the board, and community members to negotiate which problem to tackle for the COPC intervention.[27] These methods include: brainstorming, Delbecq or nominal group methods, and problem analysis (all of these are described at the end of the chapter). The Delphi method is also included at the end of the chapter and is used for consensus-building, though not for small groups. These methods enable decision-makers to work with a wide array of data such as census statistics, interviews, surveys, and focus groups (see Example 5.4).

The priority health problem may not be the one with the worst morbidity or mortality statistics, yet since it came from community consensus, it will be the problem the community is motivated to solve. Sometimes the choice of an initial intervention for a COPC project may be partly based on a community crisis. A major car crash involving alcohol, for example, may precipitate community outrage. Consider basing a COPC project on

---

EXAMPLE 5.4
Consensus Building Techniques

Narrowing a Long Initial List of Health Problems to One
Stovall, North Carolina
Author: Tom Koinis

In Stovall, NC, four focus groups were conducted to ask the question, "What are the major health problems in your community?" Members of these groups, identified mostly through local churches, totalled approximately 1% of the local clinic practice's service area. The focus groups produced a list of 21 health problems, which varied greatly with age of participants, sex, and group orientation, such as church or fire department.

Nominal group techniques were then used in a series of six meetings with a 25 member advisory board composed of volunteers from the focus groups. Feasibility criteria were established and the original problem list was pared down using nominal group techniques to four problems, one of which—access to health care for frail elderly homebound individuals—was selected to address first.

---

an issue with just such an emotional connection. The challenge is to sustain involvement in an emotionally charged problem after the acute emotion subsides. After successfully tackling one problem, the community may be more willing and able to work on other problems that aren't so emotionally charged.

After problems are prioritized, the problem analysis small group technique helps everyone involved in the COPC process understand the complexity of community problems and begin to see where they can have an impact. For example, analyzing the causes and consequences of teenage pregnancy allows the group to explore levels of the problem that lend themselves to intervention. Causes of teenage pregnancy may include low self-esteem, lack of accessibility to condoms, or lack of school-based health centers.

EXAMPLE 5.5
Prioritizing Health Problems

One Community Decides on Two Different Priorities
Sunland Park, New Mexico
Author: Frank Crespin

Sunland Park, on the Mexican border, looks much like nearby Ciudad Juarez. The community of 10,000 is among the poorest in New Mexico. Until a few years ago, it had no paved roads or public sewage disposal system.

Our health center, with collaborating agencies, began asking people of the community which health problems were the most urgent. To the staff's surprise, the top two responses were not diabetes or lack of prenatal care, but street lights and a recreation center. Without street lights people were afraid to let their children go out after dark. Without a recreation center, children turned to other ways of entertaining themselves, like drugs and alcohol.

As a participant in a funded COPC demonstration project, the health center faced a dilemma. The community wanted to address problems that would require years to solve, but the demonstration project required measurable outcomes in a short period.

Two routes were taken simultaneously: a diabetes prevention project with at-risk adults, a short-term project that could be evaluated easily, and participation in a community coalition to confront the long-term problems.

There were two lessons learned from our experience in Sunland Park. One was that health care professionals must prepare to address community health concerns that may not fit into the "medical model". The other lesson was that we must also be ready to look at outcomes that may take years to measure. In short, we may focus too narrowly on health as the absence of disease, rather than health in its broadest context. To the people of Sunland Park, health also meant safety and security. After all, what could be more important to one's health?

Methods for Task Four: Community Action Planning
Action planning is the broad process of implementing an intervention and should include the goals, objectives, strategies, resources needed, potential barriers, and timeline for each strategy. (See Appendix 5.2: Action Planning Worksheet.) Action planning can include exercises on visioning, force-field analysis, and social analysis.

A. First, identify objectives for the intervention.

B. Brainstorm criteria for strategies. Besides being feasible, measurable, and specific, strategies may have an effect on community involvement, e.g., to raise public awareness or draw in more people to participate.

C. Use the action planning worksheet to brainstorm strategies and resources. Force-field or social analysis may help you select strategies.

D. Put the strategies on a timeline and assign responsibilities.

Methods for Task Five: Participatory Evaluation
Participatory evaluation is very different from traditional evaluation in that it requires community involvement, leadership, and self-determination from the beginning. Principles include: evaluation as a shared process, co-designed by community leaders and professionals; community capacity building where evaluation skills and knowledge are transferred to community members; and an active feedback loop where community members are involved at each stage of the process.

In addition to evaluating specific interventions, evaluation of COPC processes necessarily involves understanding and measuring the development of community capacity or community empowerment.[28-30] There has been much emphasis in recent years on community coalitions and community development in the health field, but evaluations have been difficult because of the complex and evolving nature of community change. Newer publications have examined the possibilities of measuring such community capacity concepts as participation, leadership, and skill development,[31] as well as systems changes in health policy, community changes, collaborations, and civic participation structures.[32-34] Healthy community efforts have spawned the development of quality of life indicators,[35] which sometimes have included system or community participation changes as outcomes.

TECHNIQUES FOR SMALL GROUP PLANNING AND FACILITATION

Small group processes that require a minimum investment of time can be quite useful to ensure community listening, leadership development, and broad-based participation.[36-39]

Regardless of whether any particular exercise is used, each group meeting should be planned carefully. The facilitator should identify the meeting's goals and objectives before people get together. Meetings should start and end on time and follow a set agenda. Time should always be allotted for committee reports so that everyone's work is recognized.

1 Brainstorming

Brainstorming is used to gather many ideas quickly before deciding which ones to discuss in depth. Participants are asked a specific question and are encouraged to list as many answers as they can in a free-form fashion. Though it is the least structured of all the techniques, brainstorming follows two principles: the more ideas the better, and all judgments and discussion should be avoided until after the brainstorming has been completed. The latter is often difficult to control as a facilitator, because people's natural tendency is to discuss the options as they are listed. In-depth discussion of ideas can take place after all suggestions have been collected, during the prioritization of the list.

To encourage participation by everyone, the group facilitator can ask everyone to take a minute and write down some ideas before sharing them with the group, or people can divide into groups of two or three to generate ideas. During the brainstorming, one facilitator can elicit points quickly from participants and another can record them for the group to see; or one person can do both depending on the size of the group, the group members' willingness to participate, and the comfort level of the facilitator. The process often tends to build as people think of creative suggestions stimulated by others' comments.

Brainstorming can be used for virtually every community participation task, but it is less useful as a consensus-building technique because vocal people can dominate the discussion. After the list of ideas has been generated, it can be collapsed into broader categories that contain similar items. These broad categories can then be prioritized by the group using nominal group techniques.

2. Modified Delbecq or Nominal Group Technique

The modified Delbecq or nominal group technique is one of the more effective consensus-building prioritization exercises. As with brainstorming, the facilitator needs to be clear on what question to ask the group, such as "What are the most important health problems to address?" Two simple modifications of the more elaborate original technique are presented here, one for a group of up to 20 people, another for larger groups.

For groups of up to 20:

▶ Ask each person to choose his or her top three to five priorities from the list and write them on separate pieces of paper.

▶ If you want to maintain confidentiality, gather all the papers.

▶ Group them on the wall in columns corresponding to health problems. Participants will easily observe, through the length of the columns, which problems emerge as consensus priorities.

To ensure group participation, ask for someone to volunteer his or her priority health problem and ask everyone with a similar problem to bring their paper forward. Construct the columns as people participate. If there are questions whether one idea matches another, ask for clarification and a group decision on whether or not the ideas belong together. A second option is to ask people to bring forth their highest priority and see how the ideas spread out on the wall. Ask for next priorities until all columns are constructed.

For large groups (over 20):

▶ Divide them into small groups of five to seven people each.

▶ Ask everyone to write down their responses to one or more questions, e.g., what are the priority health problems? This process should be done in silence, giving people the opportunity to develop their own ideas. Consider only one question at a time and allow several minutes for people to write their responses.

▶ In each small group, individuals should then report on their ideas in a round-robin fashion, with a small group facilitator recording all responses on butcher paper.

▶ Ask each person to choose five to seven priorities, this time from the total list assembled by the small group, and rank them numerically, one for low priority to seven for high priority.

▶ Have people report their numerical rankings and record them next to each idea.

▶ Sum the rankings for each idea. The ideas with the highest rankings represent the top priorities of the small group.

▶ Reconvene the large group and ask each small group to list its top three priorities on the wall on separate pieces of paper. Combine similar priorities from different groups. You will then have an array of issues on the wall that represents the work of the small groups.

▶ Give each member of the large group a set of five colored dots and ask them to vote by placing their dots beside their top priorities—voting only once for each priority. The totals determine the large group's top priorities. People stand up and mill around until all dots are placed. This is a fun excercise.

▶ At this point, the group may want to discuss the voting patterns, redefine any terms or criteria for voting, and choose as a whole to re-rank the top prioritized problems.

The modified nominal group technique is most useful for providing everyone (providers, staff, and community members) with an equal voice in negotiating priorities. It can be used at many stages of a decision-making process, such as an early assessment of group perceptions, after a presentation of health statistics and community needs, or after deliberations on the criteria for choosing a problem. It can be used in a large town meeting or with the small decision-making COPC board. With such a versatile technique, people can develop feelings of mutual responsibility and ownership for each step of the COPC process.

3. Delphi Prioritization

Although the Delphi process is not a small group technique, it can complement the nominal group method. Consensus can be reached without convening the participant group, as follows:

▶ Administer a questionnaire to a group of experts or opinion leaders on the issue at hand.

▶ Analyze the results.

▶ Re-send the results for further prioritization if necessary.

A Delphi approach is useful when issues have already been identified, when opinions are sought from key leaders or experts who are geographically separated, and when it's difficult to arrange meetings. Statistical information can be sent with the questionnaire.

4. Problem Analysis

Problem analysis is used to develop a comprehensive understanding of the multiple causes and consequences of a health problem.

To conduct this exercise, divide a large writing surface (e.g., butcher paper) into five columns, labelled as shown in Figure 5-2. If brevity is an issue, use three columns: precursors, the health problem, and consequences.

▶ Have the group brainstorm all possible precursors and consequences of the problem as expressed within the community.

FIGURE 5.2: Problem Analysis Conducted by Community Members in Delhi, NY, To Address Teen Pregnancy

System Precursors or Secondary Antecedents	Most Pressing Precursors or Primary Antecedents	HEALTH PROBLEM	Immediate Consequences	Secondary Consequences
Inadequate education at home or in the schools Fear of parents No money No recreation for youth in community	Lack of knowledge Low contraceptive use Promiscuity	TEEN PREGNANCY	Dropout High-risk pregnancy Stress	Unemployment Increased cost of health care Teen depression

A group of interested citizens gathered in Delhi, NY, to prioritize health concerns in their community. These citizens became interested after attending or hearing about focus group meetings that the local family medicine clinic initiated to explore health concerns. The group began the meeting by prioritizing the list of health concerns generated by the focus group meetings and by results of a survey of the general public on health concerns. Using nominal group techniques, teenage pregnancy rose to the top of the list.

In the second half of the meeting, clinic leaders facilitated the group in a "problem analysis" of teen pregnancy, listing antecedents and consequences. At the end of this session, the blackboard looked like the figure shown here.

When the group then began to look at points where interventions would fit into this model, the idea of a high school clinic and improved health education was born.

▶ Discuss results of the analysis. Ask people to name the phrase or image that struck them the most. Ask what they learned about precursors and consequences.

▶ Finally, ask questions related to future actions, e.g., "Does this analysis suggest a need to reconceptualize the problem and to re-prioritize the choice of the problem for

the intervention? Are different interventions suggested
that might not have occurred before?"

Use problem analysis during action planning to test the feasibility of tackling
a particular health problem and to focus a proposed intervention strategy.

5. Action Planning

Action planning is the broad process of implementing an activity or intervention and should include goals, objectives, strategies, resources needed,
potential barriers, and timeline (see Appendix 5.2: Action Planning
Worksheet). Action planning can include visioning, force-field analysis,
and social analysis.

▶ Identify the goals and objectives for the intervention,
which could emerge as a result of the visioning exercise
or could be decided through discussion.

▶ Brainstorm the group's criteria for the strategy. Is it
feasible, measurable, and specific? Criteria should also
address the effect on community involvement. Will the
strategy raise public awareness, or draw in more people
to participate in the project?

▶ Use the action planning worksheet to brainstorm action
strategies and necessary resources. Force-field or social
analysis may be helpful.

▶ Put the strategies on a time line and assign responsibilities.

6. Visioning

A visioning exercise is often useful to balance the emphasis on problems,
build camaraderie, and develop a vision for the future that enables people
to dream beyond their day-to-day reality. One visioning exercise was presented earlier; here are others.

For a short brainstorm,

▶ Ask the group what they would like to claim as a victory
or what they envision as the best result of their efforts.

▶ Record visions on one sheet. Although the brainstorm may lead to unrealistic scenarios, it can also inspire people to imagine a wide range of creative strategies.

For a broader visioning exercise,

▶ Ask, "How would you envision a healthier community in the next five to 10 years?"

▶ Bring in markers, crayons, and paper. Ask people to take 10-20 minutes to write two columns—what they like now and what changes would express their vision.

▶ Ask people to get together in groups of four to share their visions and develop a common vision.

▶ Ask each group of four to meet with another group to merge visions. Continue re-grouping until the large group has a joint vision.

▶ Reflect on the process and outcome. Take time to examine the elements of people's visions that were not included in the joint product and acknowledge that individuals may have other goals than those expressed for the community. Discuss how to use this community vision to maintain motivation and support for the COPC process.

Visioning can be useful at various times, such as in town meetings to introduce the COPC process or with the board to develop ownership. In particular, it can stimulate creativity and expand the range of options during action planning.

7. Force-field Analysis

A force-field analysis can be used any time a group needs to analyze the forces that are promoting or inhibiting change. Put the intervention (or vision) in the center of a large piece of butcher paper and label columns as shown in Figure 5.3. Brainstorm to complete the columns, then discuss strategies to strengthen the left column and weaken the right column.

FIGURE 5.3: Force-field Analysis

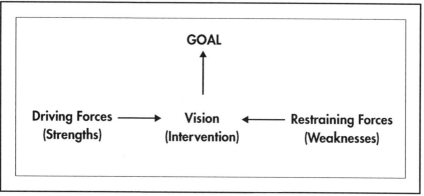

Force-field analyses can be useful when health providers are assessing their ability to engage with the community; after a visioning exercise to assess the project's ability to reach the vision; or to assess forces that may promote or hinder an intervention. For community action planning, this technique in conjunction with a social analysis provides a strategic understanding of the possibility for a successful intervention.

8. Social Analysis

The purpose of a social analysis is to strengthen community and organizational collaboration by clarifying the COPC project's position in relation to other people or organizations. Use it during community action planning.

▶ Place the name of the provider facility or COPC team in the center of a large piece of butcher paper.

▶ Ask the group to consider with which other agencies or organizations the COPC project is currently working, with which groups COPC would like to be working, and what groups, if any, are resisting the COPC process. As groups are named, place them in concentric rings around the COPC provider core, as shown in Figure 5.4.

Combine this analysis with the force-field technique to select strategies to implement an intervention and rally support. COPC efforts can be tailored to enhance existing strengths and coordinate with like-minded groups which can take over aspects of the intervention.

FIGURE 5.4: Social Analysis of School Health Project

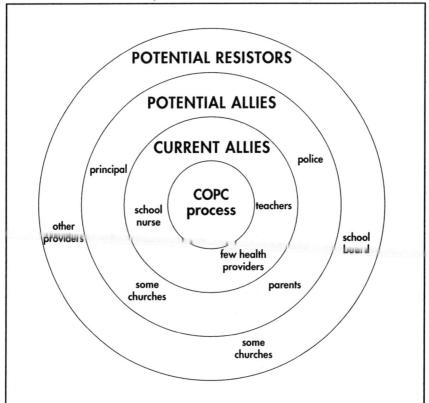

9. Focus Groups

A focus group is a marketing research technique for bringing people to-gether from a similar background to react to a set of pre-determined questions. Focus groups are basically group interviews with six to 10 people who share characteristics such as age, occupation, church, gender, or status. The facilitator prepares a list of questions, similar to an interview questionnaire, that focus on a specific topic. People discuss their answers in a free-form manner without being subject to judgment or criticism. Focus groups should take place in a neutral environment where people can feel free to express their beliefs. Some people, for example, may feel uncomfortable critiquing the health care system in a clinic setting. Facilitators should lead the group through the questions in an empathic, nonjudgmental manner, encouraging full participation.

Focus groups are useful for collecting information on health issues or community perceptions on priority health problems. They are also invaluable for planning and fine-tuning interventions, such as piloting ideas with community representatives for the intervention strategies, and pre-testing educational and media materials. Focus groups are not useful for eliciting information that people would like to remain confidential. Chapter 8 discusses focus groups in more detail.

10. Group Facilitation
Leading a group discussion that ensures full participation and decision-making is one of the most important skills in working with small groups. This skill seems easy, but can be treacherously difficult. If conducted properly, the small group can offer valuable insights and creative solutions to problems, but if conducted poorly the group can turn into an adversary or take a direction that is counterproductive to the vision or intent of the meeting. Several rules may be helpful:

- ▶ Start and stop the meeting on time to establish the expectation that participants can depend on how their time is planned.

- ▶ Establish a set agenda and follow it; allow the group to add agenda items at the beginning of each meeting.

- ▶ Ensure enough time for people to report on work done between meetings.

- ▶ Check in with the group to ensure that the discussion is staying on track; summarize the discussion periodically to make sure all participants are at the same place in their understanding.

- ▶ Use the participatory exercises described here.

- ▶ To lead discussions, prepare focus questions, such as, "What are the barriers to eliciting participation by school officials in trying to start a school clinic?"

A discussion technique that moves a group forward towards productive dialogue and decision-making is also useful. The Institute of Cultural Affairs (Technology of Participation Methods, Phoenix, Arizona) uses the acronym ORID to show the progression of questions:

▶ Ask for **objective** data, e.g., "What happened at the event?"

▶ Ask for people's emotional **reflections** on the event and their feelings or associations with present or past events.

▶ Ask people to **interpret** the value or significance that people attach to this event.

▶ Ask people for **decisions**: "What impact does analyzing this event have on our decisions for the future?"

Throughout our lives, we leave meetings frustrated because of discussions that ramble and come to no conclusion. Using ORID, facilitators can keep the discussion on track and come to a resolution.

REFERENCES

1. Goodman R, et al, eds. Community coalitions for health promotion. *Health Education Research: Theory and Practice*. September 1993; 8.
2. Minkler M, Wallerstein, N. Improving health through community organization and community building. In Ganza K, Lewis FM, Rimer B, eds. *Health Behavior and Health Education Theory: Research and Practice*. San Francisco, Calif: Jossey-Bass Publishers; 1997: 241-269.
3. Minkler M, ed. *Community Organizing and Community Building for Health*. New Brunswick, NJ: Rutgers University Press; 1997.
4. Hancock T. Healthy cities and communities: past, present and future. *National Civic Review*. Spring 1987; 86.
5. Kaufman A in Nutting PA, ed. *Community-Oriented Primary Care: From Principle to Practice*. Washington, DC: US Department of Health and Human Services, Health Resources and Services Administration; 1987;86-1:chap. 1.
6. McKnight JL. Regenerating community. *Social Policy*. Winter 1987: 54-58.
7. Freire P. *Pedagogy of the Oppressed*. New York, NY: Seabury Press; 1970.
8. Shor I., Freire P. *A Pedagogy for Liberation: Dialogues for Transforming Education*. South Hadley, Mass: Bergin & Garvey Publishers; 1987.
9. Wallerstein N, Bernstein E, eds. Community empowerment, participatory education and health - part I. *Health Education Quarterly*. Summer 1994; 21 (special issue).
10. Bracht N, ed. *Health Promotion at the Community Level*. Newbury Park, Calif: Sage Publications, Inc; 1990.
11. Wallerstein N. Powerlessness, empowerment and health: implications for health promotion programs. *American Journal of Health Promotion*. January-February 1992.
12. McMillan D, Chavis D. Sense of community: a definition and theory. *Journal of Community Psychology*. January 1986; 14:6-23.
13. Duhl L. *The Social Entrepreneurship of Change*. New York, NY: Pace University Press; 1990.
14. Nutting PA, Connor E. Community-oriented primary care: an examination of the US Experience. *Am J Public Health*. March 1986; 76: 279-281.

15. Arnstein S. A ladder of citizen participation. *Journal of American Institute of Health Planners*. July 1969: 216-224.
16. ICA. Action Planning Workshop. Phoenix, Ariz: Institute for Cultural Affairs.
17. Rivera F, Erlich J. An option assessment framework for organizing in emerging minority communities. In Tropman, J et al, eds. *Tactics and Techniques of Community Intervention*. 3rd ed. Itasca, Ill: Peacock; 1995.
18. Labonte R. Health promotion and empowerment: reflections on professional practice. *Health Education Quarterly*. Summer 1994; 21: 253-268.
19. Buchanan D. Building academic-community linkages for health promotion: a case study in Massachusetts. *American Journal of Health Promotion*. 1996: 262-269.
20. Plough A, Olafson F. Implementing the Boston Healthy Start Initiative: a case study of community empowerment and public health. *Health Education Quarterly*. Summer 1994; 21: 221-234.
21. Perkins D, Wandersman A. You'll have to work to overcome our suspicions: the benefits and pitfalls of research with community organizations. *Social Policy*. 1990: 21: 32-41.
22. Scott JC. *Domination and the Arts of Resistance*. New Haven, Conn: Yale University Press; 1990.
23. Eng E, Parker E, Harlan C, eds. Lay health advisors: a critical link to community capacity building. *Health Education and Behavior*. 1997; 24: 24-27.
24. Schiller P, Steckler A, Dawson L, Patton F. *Participatory Planning in Community Health Education*. Oakland, Calif: Third Party Publishing Company; 1987.
25. Warren R, Warren D. *The Neighborhood Organizer's Handbook*. Notre Dame, Ind: The University of Notre Dame Press; 1977.
26. Planned Approach to Community Health (PATCH). *Health Problem Identification Manual*. Atlanta, Ga: Centers for Disease Control; 1987.
27. Horowitz C, Gallagher K. In Nutting PA, ed. *Community-Oriented Primary Care: From Principle to Practice*. Washington, DC: US Department of Health and Human Services, Health Resources and Services Administration; 1987; 86-1:chap. 1.
28. Eng E, Parker E. Measuring community competence in the Mississippi Delta: the interface between program evaluation and empowerment. *Health Education Quarterly*. Summer 1994; 21: 199-220.
29. Israel B et al. Health education and community empowerment: conceptualizing and measuring perceptions of individual, organizational and community control. *Health Education Quarterly*. Summer 1994; 21: 149-170.
30. Connell J et al, eds. *New Approaches to Evaluating Community Initiatives: Concepts, Methods, and Contexts*. Washington, DC: The Aspen Institute; 1995.
31. Goodman RM et al. Identifying and defining the dimensions of community capacity to provide a basis for measurement. *Health Education and Behavior*. 1998; 25 (3): 258-278.
32. Fawcett SB et al. Empowering community initiatives through evaluation. In Fetterman D, Kaftarian S, Wandersman A, eds. *Empowerment Evaluation*. Thousand Oaks, Calif: Sage; 1996.
33. *Measuring Community Capacity Building: A Workbook-in-Progress for Rural Communities*. Washington, DC: The Aspen Institute; 1996.
34. Maltrud K, Polacsek M, Wallerstein N. *A Workbook for Participatory Evaluation about Community Initiatives*; 1997.
35. Tyler Norris Associates. *The Community Indicators Handbook: Measuring Progress Toward Healthy and Sustainable Communities*. Redefining Progress; 1997.
36. Community Tool Box: Building Community Capacity for Change, an interactive Web-based tool kit (http://ctb.lsi.ukans.edu).
37. Kaye A, Wolff T, eds. *From the Ground Up! A Workbook on Coalition Building and Community Development*. Amherst, Mass: AHEC/Community Partners; 1995.
38. Feldman M, Wallerstein N, Varela F, Collins A. *Community Organizing: An Experience for Building Healthier Communities, a Train the Trainer Curriculum*. Santa Fe, NM: Health Promotion Unit, Department of Health; 1994.
39. Norris T. *The Healthy Communities Handbook*. Denver, Colo: National Civic League; 1993.

CHAPTER 6

Defining and Characterizing Community Denominators

Tom Becker
Robert Rhyne

ABSTRACT

A COPC team needs a complete, quantitative understanding of the community in which an intervention is planned in order to measure health status before and after the intervention. Denominators can be used to measure the occurrence of specific health conditions, by calculating incidence, the rate at which new cases develop; and prevalence, the number of cases in a given population at a particular time. Many sources of information exist; they include secondary sources, which supplies data from existing studies, or primary sources, data which the practitioner collects on his or her own, an example being interviews among community residents. The US census is one of the most useful information sources for COPC. To use it, the practitioner should choose a geographic unit, or combination of units, that best represents the community, and if necessary, narrow the population to include only the denominator at-risk population of interest. Primary data collection requires great care and should be undertaken only if secondary data are inadequate for the practitioner's needs. Techniques are presented for developing questionnaires, conducting interviews, obtaining information from medical records, and studying subpopulations such as school children or employees at a worksite.

INTRODUCTION

Any medical practice today is wise to learn and employ population measurements because of the recent emphasis on managed care. Increasingly, the ability to identify clearly, assess, and measure intervention impacts on populations is an advantage for primary care practitioners in a world of shared financial risk and growing competition for primary care contracts. These population techniques enable measurement precision in discerning the impacts of interventions (a key element of COPC) and monitoring disease outcomes. The first step is learning to characterize a denominator population.

DEFINING THE COMMUNITY DENOMINATOR

The COPC process theoretically leads to the development of one or more COPC projects focusing on specific health problems or aspects of a single problem. The COPC team should select one project to start, then add projects as others are completed or as resources become available. Be careful not to overextend the COPC process by working on too many projects at once. Doing a good job on one project at a time will keep your process more manageable than doing a mediocre job on multiple projects. The process is designed to be long-term.

In conceptualizing a health problem and intervention, you may start with the broad notion of community as the residents of a geographic area (see Chapter 5) and then, using secondary data, describe the population—your community denominator. As the COPC process progresses, you will probably need to describe a subset on which to focus your intervention. For example, the project might be focused on Type II diabetes among adults in a community but later be narrowed to adults over 40, a higher risk group. The denominator you are focusing on needs to be described carefully and completely, whether it is the entire community or a subset. Several techniques exist,[1] and all have advantages and disadvantages.

Without a solid definition of the denominator population, you will not have an accurate understanding of the community in which you plan to measure health outcomes. Before you settle on a specific health problem, though, you will probably want to describe your entire community in demographic or economic terms. The project initiation team can use this information in presenting the COPC process to community groups and other health agencies that have prospective team members.

The final step is to identify a denominator that corresponds to the population at risk to develop the health problem of interest. Selection of a denominator depends on your ability to measure it accurately, the resources at your disposal, and the question you are asking. Inaccurate estimates may lead you to over- (or under-) estimate the importance of a health problem or may lead to errors in evaluating the effect of the intervention.

Denominators are determined differently for different measures of disease frequency. The two most common measures are incidence and prevalence. *Incidence* measures the rate of development of new cases—the number of new cases during a period of time (numerator cases) divided by the number of people at risk to develop the disease in the defined population over that same period of time (denominator, or at-risk population). Thus, the denominators for incidence rates include both persons and time.[2] Disease *prevalence,* the number of cases existing in a defined population at a given point in time, also requires knowledge of case numbers and persons in the population denominator. Prevalence measures are not rates and therefore do not involve time in the denominator. Their denominators include all the people at risk in a population. Prevalence reflects the proportion who have the disease at one point in time. An at-risk person has a chance of contracting the disease in question. For example, you would not count men in a measure of cervical cancer prevalence or incidence.

GATHERING INFORMATION ABOUT YOUR COMMUNITY

The two basic types of data you can use to describe the denominator are *primary data* and *secondary data*. Primary data is information *you* collect through interviews, surveys, or other means for a specific purpose, e.g., identifying the most pressing community health problems perceived by community members. Secondary data include information collected *by someone else* for some reason other than for your study. Examples include census information, state vital statistics data, and police traffic accident reports.

The type of data you will need is influenced by your stage in the COPC process. Earlier in the process, when a provider-community coalition is evolving and gaining momentum, secondary data may be adequate to help you describe the overall community denominator or gauge the magnitude of a community problem. Later, when you are designing intervention plans, characterizing a specific at-risk population, or evaluating an intervention, you will more likely need to collect primary data. You will be lucky to find a secondary source that will be useful in these latter endeavors. If a secondary data source answers exactly the same question as would your primary collection efforts, you do not need to resort to primary data collection. For example, if you decide to intervene to lower cardiovascular risk by stimulating people to exercise more, and the local health department has just surveyed your community's levels of exercise, use the health department's secondary data as your baseline.

As you may surmise, secondary data are often easier to come by than are primary data but may not directly address the COPC project. For example, when you identify a denominator population for a geographic region, census information may not correspond directly to the region you defined. You may have to estimate population demographics from the secondary census data or perform a survey yourself. Always check to see what data exist before trying to collect primary data.

SECONDARY DATA

Secondary data are available for almost every community in the country, depending on how community is defined. By far the best source of denominator data is the US census. While most other secondary data sources are concerned with mortality and morbidity, the US census provides a wealth of demographic and economic data. Appendix 6.1 lists many additional sources.

The US Census

The US census is the mechanism that defines how representatives in the House are apportioned fairly among the states; and as such is mandated in the Constitution of the United States. The census attempts to count 100% of the population and has evolved over the years into a fine technological art. Not all questions are asked of all inhabitants and therefore sampling plays a large role in the modern census.

The census provides a wealth of information in printed form, on computer summary tapes, on CD-ROM, laser discs, and microfiche. The variety of information available is shown in Table 6.1, which lists questions asked in 1990. The Bureau of the Census publishes a very useful three-part "User's Guide," available from the Superintendent of Documents (US Government Printing Office, Washington, DC 20402). "Part A. Text" covers basic information, procedures, organizations, and a detailed list of sources of information in every state.[3] This is probably the most useful of the three parts, but "Part B. Glossary" and "Part C. Index to Summary Tape Files 1 to 4" are useful if you are already familiar with the census and know exactly what you need. Also, to assist users, there are Internet pages

TABLE 6.1
1990 Census Questions

Question number	Topic or item	100 percent or sample (S)[1]		Question number	Topic or item	100 percent or sample (S)[1]	
		1990	1980			1990	1980
	POPULATION				**HOUSING**		
1	Name	100	100	H1	Coverage questions[4]	100	100
2	Household relation/ship	100	100	H2	Units in structure	100	S
3	Sex	100	100	H3	Number of rooms	100	100
4	Race	100	100	H4		100	100
5	Age	100	100	H5	Screening questions for value and rent		
6	Marital status	100	100		(acreage and commercial establish-		
7	Spanish/Hispanic origin	100	100		ments)	100	100
8	Place of birth	S	S	H6	Value	100	100
9	Citizenship	[2]S	S	H7a	Contract rent	100	100
10	Year of immigration	S	S	H7b	Congregate housing (meals included		
11	School enrollment and type	S	S		in rent)	100	–
12	Schooling completed	[2]S	S	C1	Vacancy status[5]	100	100
13	Ancestry	S	S	C2	Boarded-up status[5]	100	100
14	Residence 5 years ago	S	S	D	Duration of vacancy[5]	100	100
15	Current language and ability to speak			H8	Year householder moved into unit	S	S
	English	S	S	H9	Bedrooms	S	S
16	Age screening question (items 17-33			H10	Complete plumbing facilities	[2]S	100
	are limited to persons 15 years old			H11	Complete kitchen facilities	S	S
	and over)	S	S	H12	Telephone	S	S
17a, b	Veteran status and period of service	[2]S	S	H13	Automobiles, vans, or light trucks		
17c	Total years of military service	S			available	S	–
18	Work disability	S	S	H14	Fuels used for house heating	S	S
19	Mobility and self-care limitations	S	S	H15, H16	Source of water and method of		
20	Children ever born	S	S		sewage disposal	S	S
21a, 25,				H17	Year structure built	S	S
26	Employment status	S	S	H18	Condominium identification	S	100
21b	Hours worked last week	S	S	H19	Farm residence status	[2]S	S
22	Place of work	S	S	H20	Cost of utilities and fuels (component		
23a	Means of transportation to work	S	S		of gross rent and selected monthly		
23b	Private vehicle occupancy	S	–		owner costs)	S	S
24a	Departure time for work	S	S				
24b	Travel time to work	S	S	H21 to			
27	Year last worked	S	S	H26	Selected shelter costs for homeowners	[2]S	S
28	Industry	S	S	Derived[3]	Persons in unit (household size)	100	100
29	Occupation	S	S	Derived	Persons per room	100	100
30	Class of worker	S	S	Derived	Gross rent	S	S
31a, b	Weeks worked last year	S	S	Derived	Selected monthly owner costs	[2]S	S
31c	Hours usually worked per week last				Access to unit	–	100
	year	S	S		Air-conditioning	–	S
32, 33	Income, by type	[2]S	S		Automobiles available	(See H13)	S
Derived[3]	Family size and household size	100	100		Bathrooms	–	S
Derived	Family type and household type	100	100		Fuels used for water heating and		
Derived	Poverty status	S	S		cooking	–	S
Derived	Type of group quarters	S	S		Heating equipment	–	S
	Activity 5 years ago	–	S		Number of living quarters at address	–	100
	Carpooling arrangements	–	S		Stories in structure and presence of		
	Marital history	–	S		elevator	–	S
	Public transportation disability	–	S		Vans or light trucks available	(See H13)	S
	Weeks unemployed last year	–	S				

[1] "S" indicates sample subject covered only on the long-form questionnaire.
[2] Significantly changed from 1980 version in concept or amount of detail.
[3] "Derived" refers to items which do not appear on the questionnaire but are calculated by combining information from other items. For example, while no question specifically asks family size, family size can be determined from responses to the household relationship question.
[4] These questions help ensure that the coverage of household members is complete.
[5] Determined by the enumerators. See "For Census Use" section of the questionnaire, page 31.

on the US census, 12 regional/federal offices (see Appendix 6.2), a State Data Center program that helps 1,400 organizations nationwide provide information to consumers in every state, and a Business/Industry Data Center program with locations in many states.[3]

Defining Denominators Using Census Data
Follow the steps below when you have determined that the census method is the best way to define the COPC denominator population (see Table 6.2).[4]

▶ Choose a local agency that is responsible for disseminating census data. Part A of the 1990 User's Guide contains a complete list of data centers by state. If a local agency does not exist, contact your regional office (Appendix 6.2). Read as much of the User's Guide as necessary to complete your project.

▶ Choose geographic units for your area. If your practice area or community is geographically well-defined, use census maps and outline those areas. It usually becomes obvious which geographic census units must be used to define the entire denominator population. If it is not obvious, see the section below, "Defining a Practice Denominator."

▶ Choose variables of interest that describe the denominator.

▶ Aggregate data into the largest practical geographic units because the data are more complete and detailed for larger units. Avoid the smaller areas, where data may be suppressed for confidentiality.

▶ Narrow the population to fit a specific denominator. For example, if the project concerns falls among elderly persons, narrow the denominator population to include only persons 65 and over in the defined area. As the COPC process progresses, you may need to identify several denominators as you narrow the focus from the community to a subset at risk for a health problem.

The health problem focus will dictate which denominator needs to be developed. If practice service areas, communities, or subcommunities can be

TABLE 6.2
Developing Denominators: Steps in Using Census Data

1. Select a census data clearinghouse that can provide you information about your community.
2. Draw a line around the denominator population geographic area on a census map.
3. Choose your census variables of interest.
4. Aggregate and describe data in tables corresponding to outlined geographic area.
5. Narrow the population to correspond to a specific at-risk health problem denominator.

described in terms of well-defined geographic census units, the census is probably the best method to define denominators.

Anatomy of the Census

Two major categories of geographic areas describe the United States. The first category, legal and administrative geographic entities, includes states and the District of Columbia, congressional districts, counties and county subdivisions, incorporated places, consolidated cities, American Indian reservations, Alaska Native Regional Corporations, and voting districts. All these subdivisions have legally prescribed boundaries, powers, and functions. The second category, statistical geographic entities, includes the four major census regions (West, South, Northeast, Midwest), each containing two or more divisions defined by groups of states, for a total of nine divisions in the continental US (see Figure 6.1 and Appendices 6.3 and 6.4).

Metropolitan areas are designated by the Office of Management and Budget and meet specific population standards. Metropolitan statistical areas (MSAs) consist of cities of 50,000 or more, plus the counties where the cities are located. In 1990, there were 268 MSAs.

Urbanized areas define urban concentrations more specifically than MSAs because they consist of cities and closely related surrounding territories (suburbs) that together have at least 50,000 inhabitants. They do not include rural counties of urban centers. In fact, they can be used to differentiate urban from rural areas.

FIGURE 6.1: 1990 Census Regions of the US

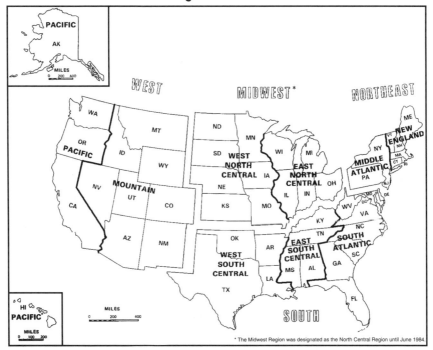

* The Midwest Region was designated as the North Central Region until June 1984.

Small geographic areas are based on counties and their subdivisions. Minor civil divisions (MCDs) are usually political or administrative subdivisions and include legally defined entities, such as towns, townships, and districts (see Figures 6.2 and 6.3). Census county divisions (CCDs) are purely statistical and subdivide counties in states that do not use MCDs for statistical data collection. MCDs were defined in 28 states in 1990. CCDs were defined in 22 states in 1990 (see Table 6.3). These county divisions can be very useful in defining denominators in rural areas.

Census designated places (CDPs) have a population density of 1,000 per square mile or greater or contain at least 2,500 inhabitants in urbanized areas. In 1990, there were 4,423 CDPs.

Census tracts are statistical areas that consist of an average of 4,000 people in counties that are generally in highly populated areas. Their boundaries do not change from census to census; thus, they provide a consistent statistical comparison. When population increases in a census tract, the tract may be subdivided, but the original boundaries are not violated. In 1990, there were 50,690 census tracts. Figure 6.3 shows a census tract

TABLE 6.3
County Census Subdivisions, 1990

State or Other Area	Counties	County subdivision		Places	
		Type	Number	Incorporated Places	Census Designated Places
Alabama	67	CCD	390	439	34
Alaska	25	Census Subarea	40	152	165
Arizona	15	CCD	78	86	93
Arkansas	75	MCD/UT	1,335	487	14
California	58	CCD	386	456	420
Colorado	63	CCD	208	267	42
Connecticut	8	MCD	169	31	86
Delaware	3	CCD	27	57	15
District of Columbia	1	City	1	1	0
Florida	67	CCD	293	390	365
Georgia	159	CCD	581	535	64
Hawaii	5	CCD	44	-	125
Idaho	44	CCD	170	200	3
Illinois	102	MCD	1,679	1,279	29
Indiana	92	MCD	1,008	566	24
Iowa	99	MCD/UT	1,656	953	2
Kansas	105	MCD/UT	1,543	627	4
Kentucky	120	CCD	475	438	33
Louisiana	64	MCD/UT	627	301	90
Maine	18	MCD/UT	530	22	84
Maryland	24	MCD	298	155	174
Massachusetts	11	MCD	351	39	192
Michigan	83	MCD	1,515	111	90
Minnesota	87	MCD/UT	2,742	854	66
Mississippi	82	MCD	410	295	29
Missouri	115	MCD	1,368	942	19
Montana	57	CCD	193	128	34
Nebraska	93	MCD	1,255	535	4
Nevada	17	CCD	67	18	38
New Hampshire	10	MCD	259	13	47
New Jersey	21	MCD	567	320	179
New Mexico	33	CCD	131	98	76
New York	62	MCD	1,013	619	350
North Carolina	100	MCD/UT	1,040	511	100
North Dakota	53	MCD/UT	1,806	366	10
Ohio	88	MCD	1,553	941	111
Oklahoma	77	CCD	302	592	6
Oregon	36	CCD	211	241	43
Pennsylvania	67	MCD	2,584	1,022	275
Rhode Island	5	MCD	39	8	19
South Carolina	46	CCD	294	270	72
South Dakota	66	MCD/UT	1,389	310	24
Tennessee	95	CCD	462	336	37
Texas	254	CCD	863	1,171	105
Utah	29	CCD	90	228	27
Vermont	14	MCD	255	51	18
Virginia	134	MCD	500	229	116
Washington	39	CCD	245	266	160
West Virginia	55	MCD	277	230	47
Wisconsin	72	MCD	1,894	583	35
Wyoming	23	CCD	71	97	12
TOTAL, U.S.	**3,141**		**35,298**	**19,289**	**4,146**
American Samoa	5	MCD	16	73	0
Guam	1	Guam	19	-	32
Northern Mariana Islands	4	MCD	18	-	16
Palau	16	MCD	19	-	3
Puerto Rico	78	MCD	899	-	220
Virgin Islands	3	MCD	20	3	6
TOTAL	**3,248**		**36,289**	**19,365**	**4,423**

county and its subdivisions. These block-by-block tracts can be very useful in defining denominators in urban areas.

In 1990 the entire nation was subdivided into Block Groups (BGs). Block Numbering Areas (BNAs) are the rural counterpart of census tracts and divide counties where there are no census tracts. BNAs represent

FIGURE 6.2: Geographic Hierarchy for the 1990 Decennial Census

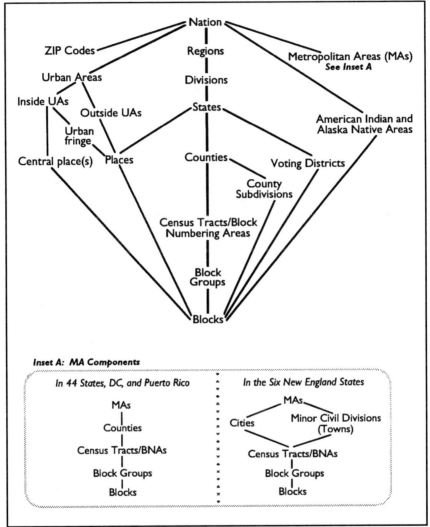

groupings of blocks within counties and are assigned specific numbers (see Figure 6.3). Block groups have the same first digit and identify specific subdivisions of counties. For Census 2000, all BNAs will become census tracts.

Blocks are the smallest census area and covered the entire US for the first time in 1990. Each block has its own number and as such is very use-

FIGURE 6.3: Small-Area Geographic Census Areas

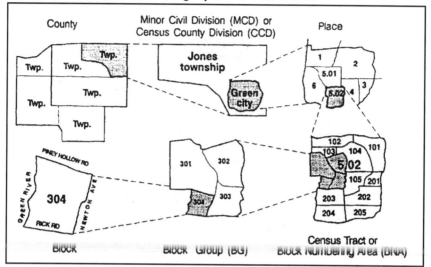

ful for COPC. Blocks are defined by streets, streams, railroad tracks, and other visible features. Also for the first time in 1990, Alaska Native village statistical areas, tribal designated statistical areas, and tribal jurisdiction statistical areas were delineated.

The relationships among these geographic units is hierarchical and can be seen in Figure 6.2 for 1990. It is important to note again that these statistical and governmental units overlap and that 100 percent of the nation's population can be represented by a combination of these different types of areas. MCDs/CCDs, census tracts, and block groups were the common principal units of the 1990 census and are the most useful tabulation units for COPC.

PRIMARY DATA

When secondary data are simply not adequate to address issues relevant to the COPC project, you will need to collect primary data, in many instances developing a questionnaire to get information from participants.

Questionnaire Development

Say you want to determine your population's attitudes about the community's most pressing health problems. The goals of your survey are to find out the basic demographics of your respondents, the community health problems they feel are most important, and potential solutions. This simple task is a potential nightmare if you are not schooled in questionnaire design, sampling techniques, and simple descriptive analyses. A large body of literature exists that examines detailed issues on asking questions and designing surveys.[5,6,7,8,9]

The first step in developing a questionnaire is defining the information you will need from each participant. Brainstorm a list of information items with your COPC team. Reflect on the list, adding and subtracting items based on your goals for the survey, your intended population, and how the information will be used. Items can include demographics, knowledge, attitudes, opinion, or any other areas. Say you are seeking the following information:

1. Differences in perceptions of community health problems by
   a) race
   b) sex
   c) age group

2. Perceptions of most pressing health problems

3. Potential solutions

Once you have a practical, complete list of variables, write a first draft of the questionnaire. Include one or more questions about each variable, more questions on each topic than you will eventually use. Organize your questions by topics and the topics by the flow of ideas you want to present to the respondent. The format of the survey, whether mailed, personal interview, or telephone, needs to be decided before the first draft is written. The advantages and disadvantages of each of these formats are discussed in the following section.

All questions must be relevant to the study's goals. Irrelevant questions cost time and money and can irritate your respondents, potentially decreasing compliance. For example, we would not include questions about ethnicity if we did not plan to examine the responses by ethnicity in our analysis. In COPC questionnaires, you may want to include a final question about the subject's interest in the project and whether he or she would be willing to volunteer or provide resources.

Make the questionnaire relevant to your audience. That means ensuring that the respondents will be able to answer the questions easily and adequately. Not only must the questionnaire meet the study's goals; the study's purpose must seem relevant to the concerns of the potential respondents. In our example above, the broad concept of "health care issues" probably will seem relevant to most community members; but a focused survey on women's health care issues or on minority health care issues may not. Ask broad questions first, then focus after you have the respondents' attention.

Fewer surveys will be completed, whether by mail, telephone, or personal interview, if the relevance of the survey is not made clear in introductory written or spoken remarks. A well-written introduction justifies the survey's goals to the respondents and stresses the importance of participation. It should briefly state its purpose and assure the respondent of confidentiality. The respondent must trust you, or his or her answers may be biased. You can use a cover page to give the introductory statement and to record time, place, date, and any other relevant information about the interview. The first draft of the questionnaire should also include clear, concise instructions for completing the questions, placed before the first question and each time the format changes.

Open or Closed Response Questions?

Closed response questions give the respondent a fixed choice of responses, whereas open-response questions ask the respondent to generate his or her own ideas. We would probably choose to ask the respondent's gender using a closed response question. But if we are asking a question that does not have a fixed set of responses or we just want to know the respondent's ideas, the open response format is better. We could ask the respondents to list the three most pressing problems facing the community. Advantages of closed category or fixed alternative questions include:

▶ Answers are standard and can be compared from person to person.

▶ Answers are easier to code and enter into a computer database.

▶ Data are easier to analyze.

▶ All answers can be completed.

▶ Respondents are clear about the meaning of the question.

▶ Answers are simpler for respondents to complete.

Open response questions could have advantages in other parts of our survey, however. For example, if we wanted to gather data or ideas about the types of interventions we could use for our community health problems, we would ask the question in an open-ended manner, i.e., "Please list the types of activities we could use to solve the health problem you have listed." Advantages are that open response questions:

▶ Can be used when all response categories are not known.

▶ Allow the respondent to answer adequately and in great detail.

▶ Can be used when there are too many potential answer categories to list.

▶ Are preferable for complex issues.

▶ Allow more opportunity for creativity or self-expression.[6]

▶ Allow for elicitation of options from a community.

Potential Pitfalls in Asking Questions

Exercise great caution in asking even the most simple question, as misinterpretation is always likely to occur, and validity and reliability of the data will be compromised. Common pitfalls include:

▶ Wording of questions is too complicated, or questions are too long. You must know something of the reading level or sophistication of the surveyed audience. Short, simple questions are preferred to long questions that contain difficult vocabulary. Generally, write your questions at a 5th grade reading level and ask yourself if respondents will understand every word.

▶ "Two-for-one" or double-barreled questions. In our example survey, we cannot ask questions such as "Are you a woman or minority?" This question actually asks two questions, and if the answer given is "yes" we do not know which question is being answered. If you really want information about both gender-specific and minority attitudes on the community's major health problems, ask at least two questions.

▶ Use of ambiguous terms. One example is "With which racial/ethnic group do you identify?"[6] Perhaps the respondent would answer that she is Hispanic if asked directly about her ethnicity, but that she identifies with African-American people because her foster parents and foster brothers and sisters were African-American. The original question would not correctly identify a person's ethnic status.

▶ Leading the respondents with "non-neutral" information. An example of such a question would be: "The community leaders think that teen pregnancy, alcoholism, and traffic crashes are the biggest health issues in our town. What do you think?" Instead, we could ask a neutral, open-ended question: "What do you think are the three major health problems in our county? Please list them below." We could also ask a more structured question: "Please rank the following 10 health problems below according to importance in the community (most important = 10, least important = 1)." Either technique avoids leading the respondents and biasing your data.

▶ Asking threatening questions, or asking sensitive questions in a threatening way. Such questions might relate to sexual preference, drinking of alcohol, etc. Placing such questions near the end of the questionnaire helps reduce some of the problems with non-compliance of the respondents. Also, you can improve response rates by assuring respondents that their answers are anonymous.

▶ Categories of responses are not mutually exclusive, allowing the respondent to have more than one correct choice. For an example of a "bad" question, the following amounts of annual income might be (inappropriately) listed as choices: $5,000-10,000, $10,000-20,000, etc. If the respondent earned $10,000, he or she could choose two responses. List the choices as $5,000-$9,999 and $10,000-$19,999, so there is only one correct response.

The order of questions is critical in achieving an acceptable response rate. Guidelines include:

▶ Warm up your respondent by asking easy questions first. In a clinic-based study of women with abnormal pap smears, we ask subjects about potential risk factors for development of cervical disease, including diet, sexual behavior, and contraceptive histories. We always begin with questions on diet, which are not considered sensitive or threatening and warm up the respondents for later, more sensitive questions.

▶ Put open response questions last.

▶ Ask information needed for subsequent questions first. In our example, we would ask for the three most pressing health care problems before asking for suggestions on how to fix them.

▶ Vary the questions in length and type to keep respondents from getting bored.

▶ Do not make the questionnaire too long. Aim for the minimum amount of time that it takes to complete the survey, while including all the necessary questions. Generally, 30 minutes or an hour is too long; 10 or 15 minutes is better. Always tell respondents beforehand how long they can expect the survey to take.

After the first draft of your questionnaire is complete, read it from beginning to end with other members of the COPC team, listing all possible misinterpretations. This is when you will find poorly worded questions, confusing questions, and other pitfalls. Revise the questionnaire, repeating the process until you are satisfied.

"The Road Test"

Once a satisfactory draft is complete, you are ready for a critical step — the "road test" or pilot test,[9] designed to spot any remaining problems and ambiguities. Administer the survey to a small number of respondents (two to five), using the same format as the final questionnaire, whether written, face-to-face, or over the telephone. Choose respondents from the target population. If possible, review the questionnaire in person with your "road test" respondents to get their feedback. If trained interviewers are to be part of the main data collection effort, include them as part of the pilot test. If necessary, shorten the questionnaire. Remember, you purposefully wrote too many questions for each item of the first draft. Revise, then perform another road test on two to five different respondents.

Pre-code items calling for closed ended responses to ensure ease of data entry. Where appropriate, include codes for "don't know" answers, "declined to answer," and missing data.[8] After assigning codes, write a coding manual with instructions for the people who join the project later and need to understand the survey data, for the people who actually code and enter the surveys into a database, and for those who perform the analysis.

Assume we have decided to administer our example questionnaire by personal interview. After we have assigned codes, our closed response questions will look like this:

"Read the question to the respondent and circle the best response to questions 1 and 2."

1. To which of the following ethnic groups do you belong?
   a. Hispanic White
   b. Non-Hispanic White
   c. Native American
   d. Other
   e. Declined to answer

2. What is your gender?
    a. Male
    b. Female

"Complete the following."

3. What is your date of birth? ___ ___ / ___ ___ / ___ ___
                                m m   d d   y y

STRATEGIES FOR COLLECTING INFORMATION

Decide upon your questionnaire's format before the first draft is written; this will dictate its wording, layout, tone, instructions, and the questions themselves. There are three possible formats: mailed (self-administered questionnaires which can also be hand-distributed), personal interview, and telephone surveys.

Mailed Questionnaires

Choosing between self-administered or personal/telephone surveys depends on many factors, including available resources, time, and projected compliance. Self-administered questionnaires have many advantages. For example, they:

▶ Are reasonably inexpensive, even if multiple mailings are necessary;

▶ Take much less energy and time to administer;

▶ Guarantee standardized wording of questions;

▶ Are immune to interviewer bias, influence, or unnecessary probing;

▶ Can be completed at the convenience of the respondent;

▶ Permit anonymity and thus encourage responses to sensitive questions; and

▶ Eliminate clerical errors by the interviewer.

Mailed questionnaires have disadvantages, however, which must be considered. Initial mailings frequently have low response rates, influenced by participants' disinterest in the topic, lack of perception of relevance, lack of ability to read, and frustration with poorly worded or ambiguous questions. Response rates may improve if you include a self-addressed stamped return envelope.

Financial incentives will probably increase response rates, but this is not always practical given the low budgets for most COPC projects. Providing even small tokens of appreciation, such as lists of emergency phone numbers, can improve compliance.

Plan in advance for potentially low return rates. Follow-up strategies include reminder letters, second and third mailings, telephone calls to non-respondents, or all three. Each adds time and expense, but it may increase the validity of your findings by increasing the response rate. Compensate for non-response by re-sampling non-respondents or increasing the initial sample size.

For example, to salvage a mailed survey that had a response rate of only 25%, we constructed a random sample of non-respondents to determine if their responses were similar or dissimilar to the respondents'. We collected their responses by telephone and compared them to the responses to the original, mailed questionnaire. We found consistent responses between groups and determined that most people did not respond because they did not think the questionnaire topic was relevant.

If you are thinking of recontacting non-respondents, make sure to code participant numbers on the questionnaires and on a master list so that you can identify the non-respondents later. To ensure the anonymity and confidentiality of your survey population, only one or two people on the COPC team should have access to the master list.

Sampling non-respondents may be too much for your project to undertake; it may be easier to adjust your sample size for an anticipated low response rate. If you need 100 responses to assure that your sampling error will be small, and you anticipate only a 25% response rate, you would have to mail 400 surveys. This strategy does not "fix" the problem of non-response bias, however, just the problem of insufficient sample size.

In addition to low response rates, there are other disadvantages to self-administered questionnaires. These include:

▶ Lack of standardized environment in which questionnaires are completed.

▶ Incomplete answers, or many unanswered questions.

▶ Inability to detect verbal and body language which might help you flag questions requiring clarification, or might spark follow-up questions.

▶ Inability to ask complex questions.

Personal Interview Questionnaires

In our example survey of attitudes toward community health problems, we may elect to identify a sample of people from patient rosters and contact them for a face-to-face interview. These interviews have several advantages over mailed questionnaires, the greatest of which is that the interviewer can ensure that all questions are answered completely and then probe for additional or clarifying information. Other advantages include:

▶ Higher response rate than mailed surveys. Persons who cannot read or write can comfortably provide answers.

▶ Non-verbal behavioral cues can help alert the interviewer that a question is being misunderstood.

▶ Standardized or controlled interview conditions.

▶ The increased flexibility of entirely open-ended interviews, allowing for spontaneous answers.

▶ A guarantee that the questions were indeed completed by the sampled respondent, rather than by a family member or someone else who may have received it accidentally in the mail.

▶ Ability to administer a more complex questionnaire than in any other format. For example, dietary histories are relatively easy to collect using personalized, face-to-face interviews. Such data are nearly impossible to collect when subjects/respondents in our clinic population are asked to complete self-administered dietary questionnaires.

Disadvantages of the personal interview are predictable and hard to control compared with mailed questionnaires. They include:

▶ Higher costs.

▶ Excessive time commitment.

▶ Bias caused by the interviewer's attitudes, gender, age, or appearance.

▶ Less standardization of wording of questions, especially in the case of open-ended questions.

▶ Potential for leading respondents.

▶ Incorrect rewording of questions by the interviewer.

▶ Interviewers consciously recording a response even when a question was not answered or asked.

▶ Less assurance of anonymity.

Our study team at the University of New Mexico has generally experienced extremely high compliance with interview questions, including high compliance on very sensitive, personal questions. Greatest success comes by repeatedly emphasizing several points.

▶ All responses will be kept confidential.

▶ Their participation is important for the community's collective health.

▶ Their participation is appreciated.

▶ There are no right or wrong answers (assuming they are telling the truth).

▶ All data will be reported in aggregate.

We also provide phone numbers and allow access to us if future questions arise, as has been the wish of our local human subjects committee.

The success of personal interview surveys depends on how well the interviewers are trained. Train them in small groups, giving them the opportunity to familiarize themselves with the questionnaire, discuss potentially difficult questions, practice administering the questionnaire (three to five times with an experienced observer/trainer), and learn to correctly record responses and ask questions.

Telephone Surveys

In our experience, the telephone interview has been grossly neglected in COPC projects. Not popular for epidemiologic studies until the 1980s, telephone interviews are now extremely common among researchers carrying out case-control studies, especially of cancer risk factors. They have many advantages; for example, telephone interviews:

▶ Can be put into place quickly.

▶ Are less expensive to implement than face-to-face interviews (perhaps 20-25% of the cost).

▶ Allow probing when indicated.

▶ Ensure adequate completeness of the questionnaire.

▶ Allow the flexibility of open-ended questions.

▶ Allow use of computer entry (directly) without the awkwardness of direct entry in face-to-face interviews.

▶ Do not involve travel.

The disadvantages of telephone interviews include:

▶ The lack of control interviewers have over respondents.

▶ Lack of non-verbal clues to help guide the interviewer.

▶ Inability to use photos or visual aids to help with responses (although such aids could be mailed to respondents ahead of a scheduled phone interview).

▶ Many people are disenchanted with telephone interviews not preceded by careful preparatory announcements, due to the flood of telemarketing calls.

Respondents' inherent distrust of telephone interviewers can be minimized, and compliance rates kept high, if the respondent is a well-known, recognized person in the community. Compliance rates may be lower, however, when sensitive questions are asked.

Random digit dialing can help you select households with eligible survey participants. The questioner usually asks to speak to a specific person in the household in order to sample a specific subpopulation, e.g., the adult who most recently experienced a birthday or the female head of household 65 years of age or older. The technique usually works by randomly dialing the last 4 digits of a phone number (pre-determined from a list), combined with the community's usual 3-digit prefix(es). Use computer software or a random number table (see Appendix 8.1), to generate the list of phone numbers. Random digit dialing is best used when the sampling unit is geographically defined. Random dialing obviously cannot be used to turn up subjects who use one medical practice, or for service areas that are not defined well geographically.

Even for community-based surveys, random digit dialing must still be used with caution, since biased data collection can result. Many households may not have phones and thus may go unrepresented, while some homes with more than one phone may be sampled more than once. Furthermore, the telephone response rate will probably be lower than with face-to-face interviews because it is easier to refuse to participate over the phone. Telephone respondents are less likely to cooperate with long questionnaires, and investigators are more likely to get inaccurate responses to certain types of sensitive questions (e.g., income levels) than in face-to-face interviews. Some media attention announcing your survey may assist with compliance, although this strategy could also introduce bias.

DEFINING A PRACTICE DENOMINATOR

Members of a medical practice might define their denominator as the community from which the active patients come.[1,2] There are no precise methods for determining the characteristics of that practice denominator, but you can estimate them by:

▶ Randomly sampling the practice population to obtain a representative geographic distribution of the patients' addresses.

▶ Plotting the sample on a census tract map, using the technique described above under "Process for Defining Denominators Using Census Data."

▶ Tabulating the demographics of the geographic practice denominator using the corresponding US census data.

An area containing approximately 85% of the sample can be defined as the practice denominator service area. The resultant descriptions can be broken down by smaller age groups, gender, and ethnic/racial groups.

Selecting a Sample

Assume you want to sample charts from a medical practice in order to estimate the prevalence of diseases in the clinic's population. Random sampling is the best way to get a representative sample; a sample of approximately 200 records provides a reasonable estimate of the practice denominator's demographic characteristics.[2]

Drawing a Sample of Charts

If your clinic's charts were numbered sequentially from one to the total number of patients, you could generate numbers from a random number table (see Appendix 8.1) and pull charts corresponding to these numbers. Most chart numbering systems are not sequential, however, and would need to be counted before sampling.[2] If your billing information is computerized, use your computer program to count and print out the total list of patients, numbering them sequentially. Then select the desired sample size, matching the number of each patient to the random numbers selected.

Or, count the charts on a single shelf where the records are stored, then multiply by the total number of shelves (assuming that all shelves have an equal number of charts). Next, compute a sampling frame by dividing the estimated number of charts by the desired sample size. For a total of 5,000 charts and a desired sample size of 250, the sampling frame is 5,000/250, or 20. Thus, you select every 20th chart out of the total of 5,000.

To begin selecting the sample, select a number between 1 and 20 from the random number table. For example, if 12 is picked, then you pull the 12th chart on the first shelf and every 20th chart thereafter, i.e., the 32nd, 52nd, 72nd, and so on.

Exclude the charts of patients dropped or transferred from the practice, patients who have moved, and patients who have not been in the office for a long time (e.g., two years). If a chart does not meet the criteria, go on to the next chart until you find one that does; then go back to your original numbering system. For example, if you find that the 32nd chart does not meet your criteria, and you must go to the 35th chart to find one you can use, the next chart you look at should still be the 52nd. In general, the number and type of inclusion and exclusion criteria will vary depending upon the purpose and subject of the study.

Extracting and Abstracting Information
Before sampling begins, decide what information will be extracted, such as name or ID number, address, zip code, age, sex, date of last visit, and any other variables you need, such as diagnoses, medications, ethnicity/race, education level, etc. These data can be used to:

- ▶ Locate patients by zip code.

- ▶ Develop a demographic and geographic definition of the community.

- ▶ Facilitate conversion of the patients' zip codes to a census tract enabling the use of secondary census data.

- ▶ Design services.

- ▶ Compare your practice population with the surrounding community to determine its representativeness.

Focus on the most useful data elements by designing a chart abstraction form that lists the information you need from each chart, with blanks next to each item to be filled in by the reviewer (see Example 6.1). Do not collect anything that you will not analyze later, but systematically organize the form so that items correspond to the order in which you review each chart. Efficiency in data gathering is an important goal.

EXAMPLE 6.1
Sample Chart Abstraction Form

Author: Robert Rhyne

Patient ID# ___ ___ ___

Wellness Center Outcomes Study
ABSTRACT FORM - Medical Chart

1. Date of review   ___ ___ / ___ ___ / ___ ___
                                                         m m   d d   y y

2. Patient medical record number (MR#)   ___ ___ ___ ___ ___ ___ ___

3. Date of birth   ___ ___ / ___ ___ / ___ ___
                                                         m m   d d   y y

Questions 4, 7, 8, and 9 involve information that may be in the medical chart. For the information requested, start with the date of the most recent medical visit before the first Wellness Center visit. End with the date of this review. Skip a date if the previous date was within 2 months.

4. Weights and Blood Pressures

	Visit Date m m / d d / y y	Weight (lbs) (round off)	SBP	DBP
a.	__ __ / __ __ / __ __	__ __ __	__ __ __	__ __ __
b.	__ __ / __ __ / __ __	__ __ __	__ __ __	__ __ __
c.	__ __ / __ __ / __ __	__ __ __	__ __ __	__ __ __

5. Were any of the following diagnoses/problems in the chart during the time of the study dates?

   Diagnosis / Problem   (CODE: Yes = 1 No = 0)
   a. Heart disease: CHF, CAD, Angina   a. _____
   b. Diabetes: NIDDM, IDDM, AODM   b. _____
   c. Hypertension   c. _____

6. Lipid Results

	Visit Date	Chol.	Trigly.	HDL	LDL
a.	__ __ / __ __ / __ __	__ __ __	__ __ __	__ __ __	__ __ __
b.	__ __ / __ __ / __ __	__ __ __	__ __ __	__ __ __	__ __ __

NARROWING THE DENOMINATOR
TOWARD PROBLEM-BASED SUBPOPULATIONS

Certain populations may be chosen for characterization in the COPC process for reasons other than their inclusion in a certain geographic area or relationship to a specific practice. This is especially useful when the COPC team gets to the phase of characterizing a specific health problem to address. Schools, employers or specific age-sex groups may be chosen because of their risk of certain health conditions, or their interest or concern about a certain health problem. When focusing on a specific subpopulation, the denominator also narrows to include all those at risk for the condition or health problem.

A defined practice or managed care population offers an excellent opportunity for the COPC team to estimate the frequency of population risk factors or health conditions. The population served by a medical practice may or may not reflect the composition of a community, but subpopulations within the practice or persons at risk for a particular health condition can provide the substrate from which to select an adequate sample for a COPC project. Most practice databases contain certain demographic and other information required for billing and claim submission, including patient age, sex, marital status, address, telephone number, employer, occupation, insurance coverage, ICD diagnosis codes, and CPT procedure codes. Most Medicare, Medicaid and other third party claims require that providers list one or more ICD diagnoses and link them to specific CPT procedure codes for a particular date of service, e.g., 272.0-hypercholesterolemia or 496-chronic obstructive pulmonary disease. The percentage of patients with particular diagnoses can be used as an estimate of community disease prevalence if you assume your patient age and sex distribution is the same as that of the community. You can check these against secondary data sources for the entire community. An obvious problem, of course, is the greater likelihood that medical practices will include a greater proportion of ill or injured persons than the community in general. Another is that many practices may not have proportionate representation of patients who have financial barriers to medical services.

Access to Special Populations for Community-Based Denominators

School Children
School children are an important subpopulation for several reasons:

▶ Schools usually enroll close to 100% of all children 6-14 years of age and a vast majority of a community's adolescents, including uninsured or poorer members in any denominator.

▶ Successful COPC interventions among school children offer many more years of potentially healthy life than among older groups.

▶ Annual data are routinely collected and may be quickly accessed.

▶ COPC interventions can be easily integrated with school activities.

Demographic data similar to those described for medical practices, health history, immunization status, screening parameters (vision, hearing, weight, height, blood pressure, etc.), and medication use can be quickly abstracted and followed over time.

Elderly
The elderly place a disproportionate burden on community health resources because of accidents, falls, chronic diseases, decreased functional capacity, and inadequate economic resources and social support systems. In contrast to school children, the elderly cannot be easily identified and accessed. Senior citizens' centers, "Meals on Wheels" programs, nursing and shelter care homes, churches, medical offices, hospitals, Medicare records, and special area surveys may have data.

Worksite
You can obtain employee demographic and health information, including in many cases screening, risk factor, and physical/laboratory data, through personnel offices or worksite health clinics, although confidentiality issues may cause a problem. COPC practitioners may wish to charac-

terize employees because of risks for particular accidents, exposures, or disability.

Hospitals and HMOs

The extensive databases at hospitals and HMOs allow you to characterize the numerator and denominator populations for problems such as major trauma, serious infections, malignancies, and cardiovascular problems that require hospitalization. Information from HMOs may include the number and type of specialist referrals, medication or ancillary services utilization rates, and ambulatory patient outcomes. Issues of "proprietary" or confidential information may pose problems; get approval from a human subjects review board.

DATA HANDLING NEEDS

The careful collection and analysis of data are central to COPC.[10] Fortunately, computers are now in widespread use and becoming ever more portable. With the addition of certain software packages, the management of your COPC projects can be made much easier than through the use of hard copy forms alone. The Centers for Disease Control and Prevention provide data management and analysis software packages at no cost, e.g., EpiInfo. This user-friendly program can be downloaded from the Internet and offers a graphics package and word processor that can be converted into data entry and data management screens. EpiInfo data sets can be read by many other, more powerful and more flexible software packages, including SAS.™[11] Other spreadsheet packages have expanded data management, analysis, and graphics capabilities. Software packages for mainframe and desktop computer use are described in detail in several publications[8] and can be compared and purchased through mail order. Regardless of what software you choose, keep backup data disks.

REFERENCES

1. Hearst N. The denominator population. In: Nutting PA, ed. *Community-Oriented Primary Care, From Principle to Practice*. Washington, DC: US Dept of Health and Human Services, Health Resources and Services Administration; 1987.
2. Zyzanski S, Galazka SS. A sampling method for defining community in a metropolitan area. In: Nutting PA, ed. *Community-Oriented Primary Care, From Principle to Practice*. Washington, DC: US Dept of Health and Human Services, Health Resources and Services Administration; 1987.

3. *1990 Census of Population and Housing (1990 CPH-R-1A) Guide.* Washington, DC: US Dept of Commerce, Bureau of the Census; 1992; pt A.
4. Rhyne RL, Kozoll R, Stewart B. Defining the practice population with census data. In: Nutting PA, ed. *Community-Oriented Primary Care, From Principle to Practice.* Washington, DC: US Dept of Health and Human Services, Health Resources and Services Administration; 1987.
5. Sudman S, Bradburn N. *Improving Interview Method and Questionnaire Design.* San Francisco, Calif: Jossey-Bass; 1979.
6. Bailey K. *Methods of Social Research.* 2nd ed. New York, NY: The Free Press, Macmillan Publishing Co; 1982.
7. Berdie DR, Anderson JF. *Questionnaires: Design and Use.* Metuchen, NJ: The Scarecrow Press, Inc; 1974.
8. Hulley SB, Cummings SR. *Designing Clinical Research: An Epidemiologic Approach.* Baltimore, Md: Williams and Wilkins; 1988.
9. Fink A. *The Survey Kit.* Newbury Park, Calif: Sage Publications; 1995.
10. Kameron DB. COPC application for the microcomputer. In: Nutting PA, ed. *Community-Oriented Primary Care, From Principle to Practice.* Washington, DC: US Dept of Health and Human Services, Health Resources and Services Administration; 1987.
11. SAS™ Institute. Cary, NC.

CHAPTER 7

Identifying and Characterizing Community Health Problems

Richard Kozoll

ABSTRACT

The first-time COPC team should start with the goal of devising a relatively brief intervention for a single issue. Health problems can be isolated at any point during their natural course; at each point, different subpopulations are affected, ranging from those at risk to those who eventually succumb. These subpopulations can be represented quantitatively as the numerator or denominator in measures of the incidence or prevalence of a particular health problem. To identify a single health problem, the COPC team creates a list of community health problems, characterizes each problem, sets priorities, then selects the most feasible problem in which to intervene. Final selection requires consensus among community members and health professionals. The team must evaluate its resources and break each problem into antecedents, consequences, and subpopulations, then evaluate possible solutions. When choosing the health problem and a feasible intervention, the team should consider the following: results of previous interventions; how much community visibility and involvement the effort will receive; sample size; data management required; and expected short- and long-term outcomes; and contingency plans for possible long-term implementation.

INTRODUCTION

At this point in the COPC process you should have thought carefully about your community and made attempts to characterize it from various secondary data sources. You may even have conducted informal surveys. Chapter 5 discusses the various levels of community participation and introduces small group facilitation methods that can be used to achieve consensus among COPC participants. Chapter 6 introduces the concepts of primary and secondary data collection, external health data, sampling, questionnaire development and survey design; skills that can be used to identify, describe and measure changes in a community population. The challenge facing you now is to focus on a set of problems that are both important and feasible to address. This chapter discusses a process which can be used to identify and prioritize problems deserving intervention on the part of your COPC team.

Because of your team's limited human and material resources, you will probably need to begin by addressing a single issue. Because of your team's need to engage and retain as much health professional and community interest and support as possible, you will probably need to choose a problem which is health-related and addressable in a relatively short time, certainly less than one year and preferably within six months. Your ultimate goal is to improve the health of your community through practical interventions.

Any health problem may take many forms and have different components that can be addressed in an intervention. A health problem may be viewed in the form of a *risk factor* before the disease actually occurs, or an *antecedent* to a disease (e.g., excessive cholesterol intake, precocious sexual behavior, smoking, inadequate recreational opportunities), a *screening finding* after the disease occurs but before symptoms appear (e.g., positive chlamydia testing, elevated blood pressure, abnormal mammogram, abnormal depression inventory found before symptoms develop), a *symptom* of the disease (e.g., headache, loss of balance, school absenteeism), a *condition* or *disease* (e.g., hip fracture, heart attack, arthritis, unintended pregnancy). A health problem can also be viewed as a *complication* or *consequence* of the disease (e.g., diabetic foot ulcer, falls, hospitalization, school "dropout," motor vehicle accident). You can be creative in identifying a health problem to address, once you realize that it can be "isolated" at any point during its natural history (see Figure 7.1). Unintended teen pregnancy, for example, can be addressed at any of the following levels: knowledge of reproductive biology (risk factor), knowledge or practice of sexual behaviors (risk factor), contraceptive use (risk factor), pregnancy (symptomatic condition), school absenteeism (complication), or need for parenting skills (complication). By thinking through health problems in this way and more carefully categorizing them, your COPC team has a better chance of reaching consensus on which component of a health problem can be addressed by an intervention.

FIGURE 7.1: The Natural History of a Disease/Condition

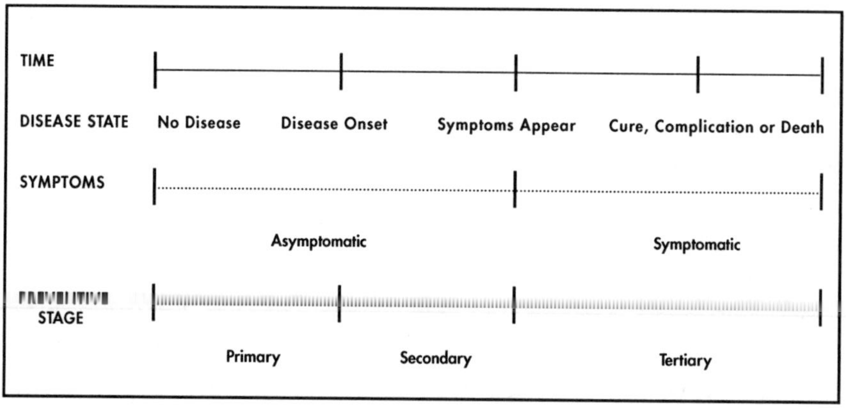

HEALTH PROBLEMS AND SUBPOPULATIONS

Each level of a health problem corresponds to a segment of the overall community population.[1] Identifying the levels of a problem also stimulates consideration of the feasibility of addressing the corresponding subpopulation. One's view of the community with respect to a health problem starts with the total community population and progressively narrows with each level of the problem from those with a risk factor, to those with the disease/condition, to those who die from the problem (see Figure 7.2).

The problem level determines which subpopulation can potentially be used as a numerator or denominator when measuring the condition frequency. These measures are usually expressed as the rate (incidence) or proportion (prevalence) of a health problem affecting a population. The denominators for incidence and prevalence measures are the populations at risk for the problem level chosen for the numerator.

Each level of the health problem can define a denominator population for your COPC project if you choose to address that aspect of the problem. The following examples use each possible level and subpopulation as a denominator for a measure of incidence or prevalence of a health prob-

FIGURE 7.2: Health Problems and Their Subpopulations

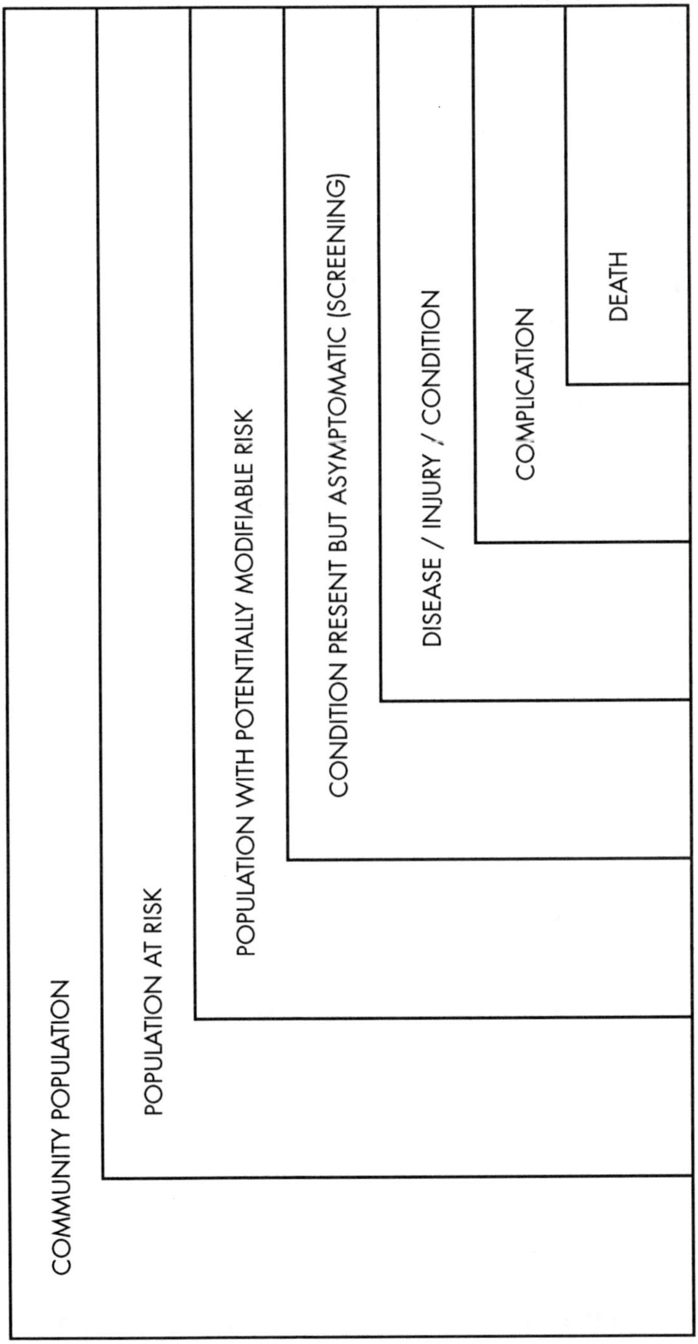

lem. Try comparing a health concern in your community to the examples presented below.

Total community population is the total population (however established) from which the COPC team is drawn. It may be the total population of a geographic area or urban neighborhood. For primary care practices, this population is the service area from which it draws its patients. For managed care organizations, it may be the total number of enrolled clients or enrollees in specific locations. The total community population is usually the largest denominator possible and can only be used as a denominator.
Examples:

▶ **Cardiovascular Disease** – Cardiac deaths per 1,000 population per year (mortality rate).

▶ **Diabetes Mellitus** – Diabetics per 1,000 population (disease prevalence).

▶ **Unintended Teen Pregnancy** – Teen pregnancies per 1,000 population per year (complication rate).

Population at risk by virtue of age, gender, or other characteristics is usually used as a denominator.
Examples:

▶ **Cardiovascular Disease** – Percentage of persons with one or more risk factors for heart disease in 1999 among all adults 18 and over (disease prevalence).

▶ **Diabetes Mellitus** – Yearly hospital admissions for diabetic ketoacidosis among Navajo children ten years of age and under (complication incidence rate).

▶ **Unintended Teen Pregnancy** – Yearly births to women 13-19 years old (condition incidence rate).

Population with a modifiable risk factor is the population subset at risk because of a lifestyle or other behavioral risk factor that can be detected before disease onset and modified by the patient, family, or medical treatment. Behavioral risk factor information is usually obtained by surveying a sample population. To determine this population, COPC projects usually face a decision to perform a new survey or extrapolate their population from other local, regional, or national survey data. This population is often used as a numerator because the modifiable risk factor can be the focus of the COPC intervention. Denominator use is also possible.

Examples:

▶ **Cardiovascular Disease** – Percentage of adults 18 and over who smoke (risk factor prevalence).

▶ **Diabetes Mellitus** – Percentage of obese children aged 10 years and under who have been screened for hyperglycemia (secondary prevention prevalence); the percentage of those with hyperglycemia (risk factor prevalence).

▶ **Unintended Teen Pregnancy** – Women 13-19 years old (teenagers) who are sexually active and single (risk factor prevalence).

Population with an asymptomatic condition is usually determined by screening a population at risk. For many conditions there is a significant period of time during which the problem is present but the affected person has no symptoms and is unaware of its presence (see Figure 7.1). This population is important because many conditions (e.g., breast cancer, preeclampsia, cervical cancer) can be more effectively treated or their complications prevented through early detection. The population that is found through screening to have such a condition is usually a numerator.

Examples:

▶ **Cardiovascular Disease** – Percentage of adults 18 and over with significant coronary artery occlusion but no symptoms (disease prevalence).

▶ **Diabetes Mellitus** – Percentage of obese children aged 10 years and under who have hyperglycemia (positive screening prevalence).

▶ **Unintended Teen Pregnancy** – Number of new positive pregnancy tests per month in women 13-19 years old who are sexually active and single (condition incidence rate).

Population with a symptomatic disease/injury/condition consists of people who are generally aware of their condition because of the presence of characteristic symptoms on one or more occasions (e.g., chest pain, excessive thirst, amenorrhea). This is usually a numerator.

Examples:

▶ **Cardiovascular Disease** – Yearly angina pectoris admissions among smoking adults aged 18 and over with no previous history of heart disease (disease incidence rate).

▶ **Diabetes Mellitus** – Percentage of children 10 years of age or less diagnosed with diabetes in a school district (disease prevalence).

▶ **Unintended Teen Pregnancy** – Percentage of pregnant women 13-19 years old who have prenatal care by the second trimester (prevention prevalence).

Population with complication(s) of a condition consists of persons who have a condition which progresses to an uncontrolled state or leads to development of an associated problem. Because prevention of the complications is often the focus of an intervention, numerator use is more common than denominator use. Tertiary preventive medicine involves this stage of the natural history of a disease (see Figure 7.1).

Examples:

▶ **Cardiovascular Disease** – Admissions for heart attack per month among smoking adults 18 and over with previously stable angina pectoris (disease incidence rate).

▶ **Diabetes Mellitus** – Cases of diabetic ketoacidosis per year among child diabetics aged 10 years of age or less (complication incidence rate).

▶ **Unintended Teen Pregnancy** – Percentage of low birth weight babies among women 13-19 years of age (condition prevalence).

Death defines the subpopulation who die as a result of the disease/condition/injury of concern. Mortality rate is occasionally used as an incidence measure and requires accurate state vital statistics death certificate information as a numerator.

Example:

▶ **Cardiovascular Disease** – Deaths from heart attacks in the US population (disease mortality rate —numerator).

▶ **Diabetes Mellitus** – Deaths per year in child diabetics 10 years of age or less (disease mortality rate — numerator).

▶ **Unintended Teen Pregnancy** – Maternal or fetal death rates among pregnant women 13-19 years of age (complication mortality rate).

Additional practical COPC uses of the concept of health problems and their subpopulations can be found in *Community-Oriented Primary Care: From Principle to Practice.*[1]

SELECTING A HEALTH PROBLEM

With the above problem and population concepts in mind, it is time to discuss the process by which your COPC team identifies an initial set of problems and then narrows the list to one problem that can potentially be addressed with an intervention. One approach of many individuals who have implemented COPC involves three sequential steps:

1. Create an exhaustive list of community health problems of interest or concern.

2. Using a prioritization process, select the most feasible problem(s) to address in your community. Characterize each of the priority problem(s) and educate the COPC team about the problems chosen.

3. Using specific criteria, choose the one problem that your COPC team feels is most feasible to address initially. If necessary, further characterize the problem in your community.

STEP 1: Create A List of Community Health Problems
The initial step in this process is to create a list of many health problems that are of current concern in your community. This process should involve collecting subjective opinion from a variety of local people and health professionals, and collecting objective data on your community from secondary data sources. Managed care concerns are also important "to bring to the table." At these initial stages you are collecting as many ideas as possible using objective data already available and brainstorming exercises (See Chapter 5 for instructions on brainstorming).

"Brainstorming" a Problem List with
Clinicians/Health Professionals/Clinic Staff
In the current environment of continuous quality improvement, liability consciousness, cost-effective management and competitive medicine, regular planning meetings are essential to the organizational structure of any practice, hospital medical staff or health agency. It is in these meetings that discussions may be most useful in achieving comfort with the integration of COPC into existing health professional systems. It is also in such meetings that one may glean from local health professionals their areas of interest and perception of community health problems. Most health professionals have experienced brainstorming during their careers; thus, participating in such a session and leading a brainstorming exercise about COPC should be an easy task for the facilitator because most will already be familiar with the process. Often the challenge in brainstorming with health professionals is to curb discussion until the appropriate time. A productive and fun brainstorming exercise at the beginning of a meeting with health professionals can help your team coalesce and set the example of an efficiently run meeting and COPC process.

Health professionals will often perceive the importance of health problems from a point of view that reflects their experience in medical practice and familiarity with vital statistics and the medical literature. A pediatrician may consider abnormal parenting to be a grave concern, while a public health nurse may identify motor vehicle accidents as most important. The intention of this exercise is to merge these perceptions and insights with those of the staff and reach a consensus on which problems are priorities.

In a primary care environment, the provider is under a lot of pressure to address acute medical problems and maintain productivity rather than devise prevention strategies. In the area of hypertension, for example, a project to assure medication compliance may seem more important to the primary care practitioners than exercise and weight control classes. Because time constraints may be such a major factor in a practitioner's level of participation in COPC, they may be very interested in the effect of COPC activities on practice utilization and reimbursement. A practitioner's interest may be heightened if the COPC project includes designing new health services through the practice, e.g., Pap smears, cholesterol checks, flu immunizations or establishment of ambulance, home health or nursing programs.

Also problematic and sometimes uncomfortable is the attempt to develop the interest of multiple providers who are competing with each other in the same community. Physicians may be more likely to agree that preventing traffic deaths is in the common interest of the community, while they may resist an effort to provide additional clinical services at only one practice location. Early recognition of and sensitivity to competing practice interests, even during initial brainstorming by one practice, will "pay dividends" with later community-wide group meetings.

"Brainstorming" a Problem List with Community Groups

The non-professional community is likely to perceive health problems from a different perspective than the health professionals. These perceptions are extremely important. Surveying the general population will often result in the identification of problems that are not strictly medical or even health-related, such as transportation, poverty, lack of health insurance, low self-esteem, etc. Community leaders may be occupied with such problems as unemployment, community services, and their own political agendas. When asked to prioritize health problems in their community, people may be inclined to list these complex social problems that, although related to health consequences, will often differ from the more specific health problems listed by primary care practice personnel and other professionals. While social problems and health problems are certainly inter-

EXAMPLE 7.1
Creating a List of Community Health Problems

Stovall, North Carolina
Author: Tom Koinis, Jenny Koinis

Stovall's process of building a community team used focus groups, team building, brainstorming, and nominal group techniques.

In preparation for the first Community Advisory Group meeting, the project coordinator met with 281 people at 15 different community and church focus group meetings and conducted nominal group techniques to prioritize health problems and enlist volunteers for the group. Twenty-five advisory group members were enlisted for the Community Advisory Group. At their first meeting, they divided themselves into four small groups (by "counting off") to further consolidate and narrow the "long list" of community health problems identified through the focus group meetings into a "short list" of problems from which a project could be developed.

The following is a list of problems identified in brainstorming sessions and focus group meetings (ranked from most frequently to least frequently noted)

1. High cost of medical care
2. Illegal drugs
3. Home health care/caregiver education
4. Hypertension
5. Alcohol
6. Diabetes
7. Care of frail/poor seniors
8. Cancer
9. Heart disease/attack
10. Lack of exercise
11. Doctor's house calls
12. Cost of medicine
13. Transportation to health care
14. Teen pregnancy
15. Diet/fast foods
16. AIDS
17. Cholesterol
18. Obesity
19. Day care for the young
20. Stress/children's stress
21. Teen sex problems
22. Filthy garbage
23. Child abuse and neglect
24. Smoking
25. Mental illness
26. Care of the disabled
27. Abuse of prescription drugs
28. Alzheimer's and aging
29. Lack of knowledge in health care
30. Screenings
31. More specialists per doctor

related, COPC usually focuses on specific health problems because they are more familiar territory and can be addressed on a scale that can show results more quickly. This should not necessarily dissuade a COPC team from addressing more complex social problems; certainly there are many strengths of the process that can be used to successfully approach these larger social issues. However, your team may wish to consider an initial level of focus which will lead to interventions that can be more quickly completed and best commit COPC teams, practices and communities to the process.

The aim of the brainstorming session is to generate a complete list that can then be whittled down using a prioritization technique (see Example 7.1). A critical activity that may be accomplished simultaneously with the brainstorming of potential health problems is the identification of community members who are willing to work as COPC team members. The success of the COPC team may depend on building a team with broad-based community representation who can work well together.

STEP 2: Prioritize Health Problems And Educate The COPC Team
Prioritization of a List of Health Problems
As has been mentioned repeatedly, it is worth your team's effort to focus its initial efforts on one problem. Following various brainstorming efforts, the COPC team will meet again to consider the results. The lists from health professionals, community groups and any other brainstorming exercises should be presented by representatives from each of the groups and combined into one complete list. Problems surfacing from the team's review of objective secondary data can also be added to the list.

At the first and each subsequent team meeting, experts and resource information (i.e., objective data such as surveys, maps, and statistics) should be available for educating the team about specific problem areas. Everyone should be made aware from the beginning about limitations such as funding, geographic constraints, and time frames. Tension arising from differences of opinion will need to be addressed through sharing common goals (i.e., improving the community's health) and group prioritization processes that include all participants.

The objective of the first team meeting might be to perform team building exercises and to get everyone's views on the table. After orientation and presentation of the results of previous brainstorming meetings any additional health concerns should be added to the list using a brain-storming exercise with the entire team. Conducting this exercise will en-

---

EXAMPLE 7.2
Prioritizing the List of Community Health Problems

Stovall, North Carolina
Author: Tom Koinis, Jenny Koinis

In order to consider the feasibility of each potential area listed in Example 7.1, a list of six questions was developed which was answered for each area. These included:

1. How many people would it involve?
2. Is it health related?
3. Proposed time frame?
4. Dollar cost and personnel cost?
5. Group interest?
6. What do we need to know to do project?
7. What would be measured?

The list of priority problems (the short list) after prioritization and feasibility assessment was

1. Substance abuse
2. Transportation to Stovall Medical Center
3. Elderly homebound caretaker education
4. Hospice care
5. Eligibility worker at Stovall Medical Center
6. CPR education
7. Hospice "van" for rural areas

Through further COPC team meetings, the problem of resources for frail homebound elderly was decided upon as the focus of the first Stovall COPC project, and a project addressing their needs was undertaken.

sure that all team members have had the chance to express their views on health problems. This will also ensure that everyone starts out on the same level of involvement in the process.

Reaching consensus on a shorter prioritized list of problems is the next step (see Example 7.2). The setting for consensus building should be conducive to uninterrupted discussion, be as non-stressful as possible, and the meetings should be scheduled with sufficient protected time for discussion. The group will need to meet under circumstances conducive to consensus building and at a time convenient for maximum participation, usually during a weekend day or weekday evening. It should be in a convenient neutral location that is non-threatening and comfortable for all participants. The room should be equipped for open discussion by everyone. Recording and displaying equipment such as blackboards or flip

---

TABLE 7.1
Feasibility Criteria for Selecting a Health Problem

1. Previous Successful Interventions
   a. Literature review
   b. Talk to others who have tried it

2. Community Acceptance
   a. Visibility
   b. Resources
   c. Involvement

3. Intervention Strategy
   a. Intervention Subpopulation
   b. Intervention Design
   c. Sample Size
   d. Measurable Outcomes (Variables)

4. Data Management

5. Long Term Implementation

6. Resources Available to Address the Problem

---

charts, markers and masking tape should be readily available. Neutral seating arrangements are helpful, i.e., in a circle, and a facilitator should

be identified who will encourage participation by all. You should anticipate several meetings to educate yourselves and reach a consensus.

Up to this point most of the suggested problems may have come from
opinions of health professionals and community members. Now is the
time to answer the questions such as: Do the problems suggested by opinion agree with the more objective information from secondary data? Does
a problem look feasible for your team to address? Is there sufficient health
professional or community interest to sustain an intervention? Are there
controversial aspects to addressing a problem on a community level?

If your team is discussing a particularly involved set of issues, a re-
treat using an experienced facilitator may be the preferred setting for your
first several meetings. At this point you will probably have your core of
health professional and community people, along with new members
"picked up" through brainstorming exercises and other practice and community involvement. A nominal group technique (see Chapter 5 for details) should be used to prioritize the list of problems generated from the
brainstorming exercises.

Once the priority list has been generated, the team should discuss the
reasons why people listed these specific problems as their top priorities.
In this first round of discussions that follow this prioritization process, it
will be apparent where there is agreement, where there is disagreement,
and where there should be education regarding the issue being discussed.

Next, criteria can be used to assess the feasibility of an intervention
addressing each higher priority health problem. The purpose is twofold:
to identify additional learning issues for COPC team members and to re-
rank problems after assessing feasibility of addressing them at the community level. Table 7.1 lists these criteria and they are discussed in detail
below under Step Three. Many COPC teams choose to generate their own
criteria (See Examples 7.2 and 7.3), and those in Table 7.1 are offered to the
reader as just one approach.

Every effort should be made to address each problem on the top of the
priority list using objective resources, where possible, to educate the team.
The goal is to collapse the list to fewer and more workable categories and
problems. It may be helpful for participants to know beforehand who has a
particular stake in a problem being discussed, and who the supporters and
opponents are to any and all of the prioritized health problems.

EXAMPLE 7.3
Prioritizing Health Problems

A Suburban COPC Team Uses Five Criteria to Select a Problem
Boston, Massachusetts
Author: Suzanne Cashman

A group of agency and lay people who were interested in improving the health of their suburban town began meeting once a month with the local health officer and staff of a COPC training program. A community hospital interested in reaching out to this community had provided partial financial support for the program to provide leadership in applying COPC in this community. Constituted as an advisory health planning body that would manifest the principles of a community-professional partnership, this group focused their efforts on carrying out each of the steps of COPC. At their eighth meeting, the group was ready to set priorities on the health issues that they had identified through a variety of data gathering efforts. To set priorities, they used a technique that the Director of the Health Resources and Services Administration presented in a 1989 American Public Health Association meeting. The value of this approach is not so much in its apparent precision, but rather in the specificity of factors that it articulates, most notably including public concern as a separate criterion. The technique asks people to consider five parameters for any issue as they set priorities. Each parameter is rated along a continuum of 0 (low) to 3 (high). The parameters are: magnitude of the problem or issue, severity of the problem or issue, efficacy of prevention, efficacy of treatment, and public concern. Displayed for example are several of the health care issues the group considered and ranked:

The facilitator must also be prepared to help the team through the consensus process to achieve a feasible project. Once the discussion has covered as much background on educational learning issues as is necessary,

	Magnitude	Severity	Prevention	Treatment	Concern	Total
Asthma	1	2	2	3	2	10
Alcohol/ Drug Abuse	3	3	1	2	3	12
Youth Alcohol/ Drug Use	1	1	3	2	3	10
Teen Smoking	2	1	3	1	3	10
Cancer	1	1	1	2	2	7
AIDS	1	3	2	1	2	9
Angina	1	1	2	2	1	7
Bacterial Pneumonia	1	1	2	3	1	8

After the planning committee members had tallied the totals for each of the problems/issues that had been identified, they discussed the resulting rankings and their implications. The discussions were quite intensive and lengthy, but the planning committee felt it was important for all members of the group to have a chance to express their thoughts regarding the choice of a problem for intervention. Additional aspects of the decision that entered the discussion at this point were the resources needed and potentially available to develop and implement an intervention, as well as consideration of which issue/ condition most lent itself to a successful outcome. The goal was not only to select a problem/issue, but to build consensus and buy-in among all members of the group. This process contributed to the development of the nascent community-professional partnership. Ultimately, the issue of youth alcohol and drug use was combined with teen smoking to become "youth risky behaviors," the topic the committee selected as the first issue they would begin to address.

the team should again engage in a consensus building process as described in Chapter 5.

Educating the COPC Team

After the priority list has been established, and before the health problem has been chosen, COPC team members should educate themselves about the specific problems being considered. Every team member should learn enough about the high priority problems so that he or she feels sufficiently informed to independently assess the feasibility of addressing them. During this education phase the participants should explore information about the community's health problems from sources such as those listed in Appendix 6.1. Analysis of the problem may include breaking it down into its various levels of antecedents and consequences as discussed in Chapter 5 under problem analysis techniques and in the introductory material in this chapter. Health professionals in the community may also be a valuable resource for educating the COPC team about the prioritized problems being considered.

STEP 3: Choose One Health Problem that Your Team Agrees is Feasible

At this point in the process the COPC team will have:

- ▶ Generated a long list of potential health problems that have been identified by brainstorming exercises and secondary data sources.

- ▶ Undergone some type of nominal group prioritization technique that has resulted in a short list of high priority problems.

- ▶ Performed a problem analysis on the top priority problems, breaking down each problem into its component parts (antecedents and consequences) and subpopulations.

- ▶ Educated its members about the top priority problems and potential solutions.

The next step for most new COPC teams will be to select the initial problem and intervention.

The process of choosing one health problem and planning a feasible intervention usually cannot be done separately. Use the feasibility criteria below to accomplish the two tasks simultaneously (see Table 7.1).

1. Previous Successful Interventions

How have other people designed interventions to deal with the health problem you are considering? Someone else has probably attempted to address the problem you are considering and hopefully has written about their experience. It will be time well spent to look at the success or failure of approaches others have taken in addressing the problem. You can approach this by performing a review of the literature and/or talking to those who have designed interventions to deal with issues such as those identified in your community. The results of interventions that didn't work well are less likely to be published than the results of interventions that did work well. If published, the areas that gave the authors the most difficulties may not be fully described in their writing. Therefore, it can be helpful to talk to them directly.

The choice of an intervention that has a "track record" of success elsewhere and is appropriate to the health problem of concern will maximize your chance of success. Review the US Preventive Services Task Force assessment[2] and the current literature in the context of the problems you are considering.

2. Community Acceptance

a. Community Visibility

Your initial COPC intervention may need highly visible results in order to establish the presence of and gain support for COPC in your community. Will your initial intervention give you the visibility you need? Can your team coordinate or collaborate with other individuals and agencies working on the same or similar problems? Can you avoid "territorial issues" that may detract from community acceptance of your effort?

b. Community Resources

Are the COPC team and community people associated with the COPC project able to carry out the proposed intervention? How long is it likely to take? Would an easier and quicker project be better? For example, if your team is considering a smoking intervention and want smoke-free public buildings, can you accomplish this goal? Will it take longer-term legislative or regulatory action? If a voluntary effort is attempted, do you have the time and people to work with individual businesses and offices?

How much training and supervision will they require? Would it be easier and quicker to sponsor a smoking cessation intervention?

c. Community Involvement
Your team may need to choose an initial problem or intervention that will engage more community people and quickly reinforce the commitment of those already involved. Will the problem and intervention under consideration lend itself to this need? If your team has chosen to address adolescent drug use with an alternative recreation program, how many community people or professionals are likely to participate? Will your team be likely to experience some quick gratification or early successes to reinforce its continuing effort?

3. Intervention Strategy
Is the intervention likely to work? How soon will you know if it is working or not? How quickly do you need to know the results of the intervention? If your team proposes to increase childhood immunization levels, will a community-wide tracking system linked to all health care providers accomplish the goal? How many months (or years) will be required to determine if immunization rates are rising? Four critical aspects of intervention planning are suggested below for consideration.

a. Intervention Subpopulation
Who is expected to benefit from the intervention? Can you define the specific subpopulation that corresponds to the problem and intervention you are proposing? (See Figure 7.2.) If your intervention requires "client or patient enrollment," who will be eligible? If the intervention is a community-wide education program, what group will be assessed for change in knowledge, attitude or practice?

b. Intervention Design
The more simply and clearly your intervention can be understood and carried out, the more likely it will succeed. If you are addressing suicide risk, how will you deal with antecedents such as a recent loss, depression, drug use, etc.? Do most people in the community understand such relationships? Do all members of your COPC team understand them? Is there a universally understood and accepted approach with which to address the risk

factor(s)? If you are working with a group of people, will it be necessary and/or feasible to have a control group for comparison? If not, how can you detect changes in the intervention subpopulation? Various study designs which may be applicable to COPC projects are discussed in Chapter 8.

c. Sample Size

How many people should be the focus of your intervention? Will you have sufficient numbers to show a beneficial effect? There are two major factors to consider, effort to intervene and effort to measure. "One-on-one" interventions (e.g., an aerobics class) are resource intensive, and therefore can involve only a small percentage of a subpopulation. Media health education, on the other hand, requires less intervention effort, but will usually entail some sort of survey sample to measure the results. With some interventions the potential sample size is limited because the subpopulation is small (e.g., DWI offenders). Will this be a problem in designing an intervention or measuring its success?

If you are going to perform statistical testing to determine the effect of your intervention, you should estimate the required sample size before you start. There are many books and computer programs available to assist you.[3-9] The procedures for estimating sample size are different depending on which data analysis methods you will use. Some of the commonly used methods are discussed in Chapter 8.

d. Measurable Outcomes (Variables)

What are the expected short-term or long-term outcomes of the intervention? How will you know "when you have them?" COPC requires an ongoing cycle of measurement and adjustment. You will need to choose measures appropriate for the problem and understood by the community. For example, if you institute a smoking cessation program among reproductive age women, a short term outcome might be percentage of smokers who quit. A longer term outcome might be the reduced incidence of low birth weight babies in the community. Which you choose may depend upon how long you intend to intervene, and which variable can be best understood by the community.

4. Data Management

How much effort and resource will it take to gather the necessary information to assess your intervention? How far do you need to go with collecting, processing and analyzing data to be reasonably certain your intervention is working? A convenient approach is to gather evaluation data during the normal course of the intervention. Can this be accomplished, or will there have to be a special survey or other procedures to gather the information? For example, if your intervention involves a "road-block" to distribute seat belt use information, you could perform an "on-the spot" survey while handing out a pamphlet. If your team decides to organize a community-wide exercise promotion campaign, you may need a special survey to ascertain exercise habits.

Data management issues that often arise include survey design, manual versus computer data processing, procedures for analysis, and organization of data for team and community presentations. If your team does not consist of persons with experience in these areas, you may wish to consider outside consultation from a community agency, health authority, or educational institution. Experts with these organizations are often gratified to be included in a COPC effort and may become a "standing resource" for the team.

5. Long Term Implementation

A common experience is for a COPC intervention to continue for a time period long beyond that anticipated, or to "lose momentum" before its anticipated conclusion. This may reflect the important and difficult community-wide problems that are often chosen for COPC attention.

If an intervention is "working," and community interest remains high, it is often wise to "pass off" the project to an agency that has the interest and resources to sustain the effort. For example, a local managed care organization might be able to maintain a high-risk prenatal tracking program and monitor the incidence of infants with perinatal problems in the community.

If, on the other hand, an intervention is "not working" or community interest and commitment are waning, a COPC team will need to determine if the intervention can be modified, the problem addressed another way, or the project terminated and attention was diverted in another direction. Such decisions often require skill on the part of team leaders to maintain committed individuals on the team and in the community. It is often helpful for the team to adopt a philosophy of analyzing and learning from each effort, regardless of its perceived success.

6. Resources Available to Address the Problem

A common experience on the part of COPC teams is to underestimate the human and financial cost to carry out implementation and evaluation of an intervention. After a plan has been proposed, an initial effort should be made to "cost it out." This will often lead to a preliminary decision to eliminate the plan or seek outside resources (e.g., a grant or contract) to carry it out. Persons familiar with potential outside funding sources are usually available in regional or state agencies, and should be approached when necessary. In addition to agency officials, faculty at colleges and universities or students who may be interested in community projects are often gratified to assist, and can also become "standing resources" for the team.

ONE LAST TASK:
FURTHER CHARACTERIZING THE CHOSEN HEALTH PROBLEM

At this point, your COPC team has chosen the most suitable problem for focusing its next efforts. In the process of prioritizing and selecting it, your team has most likely gathered considerable expertise and may have a specific subpopulation, intervention, and measurement plan in mind. Now revisit the concept of measurement and ensure you have a valid and feasible method for characterizing the problem. In many if not most cases, your initial characterization method will serve as the first and subsequent measurement of your intervention success. Your major choice will be to utilize secondary data sources (e.g., vital statistics, hospital/clinic reports) or collect primary information in your community.

If your team chooses to perform a survey (as many do), you will probably interview and possibly take physical or laboratory measurements from individuals. Your dilemma will probably relate to whether to choose a "convenience" sample (e.g., health fair attendees, Saturday shoppers, etc.) because of its ease and low cost or engage in selection of a more random selection of people who are more likely to reflect the true situation of the at-risk population. If your initial characterization is also your baseline measurement for your intervention, you may wish to lean towards a more rigorous method of random sampling.

Many secondary data sources are available to characterize your problem on a local level. (See Appendix 6.1 for additional information.) Hospital records, office records, school health records, vital statistics, and insurance claim data are all useful resources. Confidentiality issues, although important, can usually be surmounted with a little local creativity. Hospital records can be a rich source of information about the incidence and prevalence of health problems and their complications and can also be used for primary data collection. A hospital "face sheet" or discharge summary will contain a principal diagnosis (i.e., the condition for which the patient required hospital care) and several other diagnoses or complications often sequenced in the order of their importance. It will also list therapeutic procedures performed. The physician's admission history and physical examination will typically contain more detailed information about the patient's underlying conditions, risk factors, and circumstances of presentation to the hospital. The daily progress notes and discharge summary will provide information about the condition requiring hospitalization and the course of treatment. If only face sheet information is needed, the hospital's computer data base may obviate the need for individual record review.

Physician's offices and clinics can also provide a rich database on health problem information. If one office or clinic's patient population will not accurately reflect the entire population at risk, data will often have to be abstracted from more than one site and aggregated for use by the COPC team. Offices and clinics offer the opportunity for prospective as well as retrospective data gathering. An example of prospective data collection would be collecting information on dietary compliance from each diabetic patient as he or she comes in, using a standard abstract form. Prospective efforts, however, require a certain level of commitment and effort from individual health professionals and office/clinic staff who may not be part of the COPC team.

School nurses typically maintain records on each school child which contain key information such as immunization status, screening test results, and chronic conditions requiring ongoing medical attention. This information can be accessed retrospectively or prospectively and may be summarized at the end of the school year for educational authorities. Summary information (if you can wait for it) may represent a convenient short cut for characterizing certain health problems of school age children. Be sure to go through the proper channels to gain access to these records. And, remember, confidentiality is of utmost concern.

Vital statistics include birth, death, and pregnancy and other maternal and child health information which is usually collected and published by state departments of health. If a unique data summary (e.g., a multi-year period or sub-county geographic area) is needed, state agencies are often able to accommodate a special request. State or county health departments also may have statistical information, and they participate in a national behavioral health risk factor survey which collects ongoing health risk information from randomly selected telephone respondents. This information may also be accessed to characterize a health problem of concern by your COPC team.

Claims data from Medicare/Medicaid fiscal intermediaries, managed care organizations, insurance companies, and employer-funded health plans may also be useful for problem characterization. These organizations may be particularly responsive when informed of the purpose and principles of COPC. In the emerging environment of managed care, organizations are very interested in developing ways of tracking outcomes data and preventing disease. Community involvement and visibility are often as much in their interest as they are to the COPC team.

Although of limited usefulness for COPC efforts, national data pertaining to births, marriages, divorces and deaths are available from the National Center for Health Statistics and have been analyzed in terms of national health priorities by Rice.[10]

The United States Department of Health and Human Services on September 5, 1990, released national health promotion and disease prevention objectives for the year 2000.[11] There are 297 objectives organized into 22 categories based upon health problems, and within each category are three classifications:

▶ Health status ("HS") objectives,
▶ Risk reduction ("RR") objectives, and
▶ Services and protection ("S&P") objectives.

Specific problems (including risk factors) within each classification are quantified, and reduction targets are set as a national health priority. Review of these problems and reduction targets may be very helpful to

COPC teams in selecting local problems and developing measurable objectives for each.

National resource lists corresponding to each health problem category outlined in *Healthy People 2000: National Health Promotion and Disease Prevention Objectives* have been developed by the Office of Disease Prevention and Health Promotion of the Public Health Service, US Dept. of Health and Human Services, and are included in the appendices of that publication.[11] Invaluable national data and intervention suggestions can be obtained by contacting the agencies listed.

An unusually thorough analysis of health problems of the elderly, including national baseline data on specific problems and a detailed list of references was published by Stults[12] and is recommended to any COPC team contemplating an intervention with this population. And as mentioned, the US Preventive Services Task Force[2] has assessed the effectiveness of many preventive interventions. Baseline information on underlying health problems termed the "burden of suffering" along with a summary of available national data on intervention effectiveness and feasibility is well worth reviewing in the context of problems identified by COPC teams.

The characterization of an initial health problem marks a major accomplishment for the COPC team. Up to this point, the efforts have been somewhat general, but now they are focused on a specific problem. The subpopulation denominator has been identified and the extent of the problem in that population has been assessed and measured. This initial characterization is important because it is the most vigorous measurement of the problem so far in the COPC process, and it establishes a baseline against which you can compare subsequent measurements to determine if the intervention you have chosen has an impact.

REFERENCES

1. Kozoll R. A health problem characterization schema using sequentially smaller measurable populations. In: Nutting PA, ed. Community-*Oriented Primary Care: From Principle to Practice*. Washington, DC: US Dept. of Health and Human Services, Health Resources and Services Administration; 1987.
2. US Preventive Services Task Force. *Guide to Clinical Preventive Services*. 2nd ed. Baltimore, Md: Williams & Wilkins; 1996.
3. Cohen J. *Statistical Power Analysis for the Behavioral Sciences*. 2nd ed. Hillsdale, NJ: L. Erlbaum Associates; 1988.

4. Duncan RC, Knapp RG, Miller MC. *Introductory Biostatistics for the Health Sciences.* 2nd ed. New York, NY: John Wiley and Sons; 1977.
5. Kraemer HC, Tiemann S. *How Many Subjects? Statistical Power Analysis in Research.* London, England: Sage Publications; 1987.
6. Borenstein M, Cohen J. *Statistical Power Analysis: A Computer Program.* Hillsdale, NJ: Lawrence Erlbaum Associates, Inc; 1988.
7. Zar J. *Biostatistical Analysis.* Englewood Cliffs, NJ: Prentice-Hall, Inc; 1974;577.
8. Hulley SB, Cummings SR, eds. *Designing Clinical Research: An Epidemiologic Approach.* Baltimore, Md: Williams & Wilkins; 1988.
9. Rice DP. Health status and national health priorities. *West J Med.* 1991;154:No.3.
10. *Healthy People 2000: National Health Promotion and Disease Prevention Objectives.* Washington, DC: US Government Printing Office; 1990. DHHS Publication No. (PHS) 91-50212.
11. Stults BM. Preventive health care for the elderly. *West J Med.* 1991;141:No.6.

CHAPTER 8

Evaluating Your Intervention

Deborah Helitzer
Robert Rhyne
Betty Skipper
Laurie Kastelic

ABSTRACT

To design an intervention, the COPC team first writes a detailed plan specifying objectives including population, desired change, time frame, participants' roles, design, and how change will be measured. The team then lists necessary resources and any other constraints. To implement the design, the team needs a system for assigning tasks, implementing a marketing plan, conducting the intervention and collecting data. Like the intervention plan itself, the marketing plan should include goals, the specific information to be conveyed, lists of potential marketing strategies and resources, and evaluation criteria. Sample components, outlines, and phases for implementing and managing an intervention are presented. COPC evaluations should document both process and outcome and may use quantitative methods and/or qualitative methods such as focus groups, in-depth interviews, and participant observation. Evaluation data must be rigorously transcribed, coded, summarized, and analyzed to determine the impact of the COPC project, and teams can use the information to improve their programs. The authors discuss methods for classifying, managing, and analyzing quantitative and qualitative data, designing evaluations, and determining sample size.

INTRODUCTION

The intervention is the hub of the COPC process. It can be defined as the specific program designed to change health behaviors in a community setting. It is the mechanism by which you reach your ultimate goal of changing health behaviors and improving a community's health status. The experience of having planned, implemented, and evaluated an intervention enables the team to learn valuable lessons about the process, lessons that can help improve subsequent COPC efforts. If successful, the intervention can be incorporated into the community's health care system; if not, the COPC team can turn its attention to another problem in the community or try another intervention on the same problem. But how do you know if the intervention does what it was planned to do, change behaviors? How do you know if the intervention was even implemented as you planned?

The only way to determine if your intervention has been successful in changing behavior is to evaluate it. And, the only way to determine if your program is being implemented as you intended is to evaluate it. Your evaluation will also help you document that the strategies and activities you designed are being implemented and whether or not you achieve the objectives you set out for yourself.

PLANNING YOUR INTERVENTION

Once you have assembled the COPC team, organized a community support effort, characterized your overall community and generated a list of potential community health problems to address; it is time to turn your attention toward the details of potential intervention programs. In Chapter 7 we discussed the process of narrowing the list of health problems to one that will be the focus of an intervention. The steps used in identifying a health problem also help you design an intervention.

Pay attention to detail when planning and implementing the intervention; its success depends upon the thoroughness of this planning stage. The intervention program has two steps:

> ▶ Write a detailed plan, specifying measurable objectives, which then serves as an implementation and evaluation guide. The planning document can also be used to familiarize people with the project specifics and to answer questions that may come up among COPC team members

during the intervention. As problems are solved, the written plan can be updated. (Put a revision date on all drafts.)

▶ Implement the design. Devise a system for managing the program, assign tasks, implement a marketing plan, conduct the intervention, and collect data to evaluate it.[1]

Writing the Plan

Planning the intervention is an extension of the strategic planning model (see Chapter 4). The components of an intervention plan correspond roughly to steps of the strategic planning process.[2] In this discussion we assume that each component of the plan is developed with COPC team consensus, as discussed in previous chapters.

The **goals** statement should state what you expect the intervention to accomplish and should specify the at-risk subpopulation, the specific behaviors or health problem to be addressed, and the magnitude and direction of change expected to result. **Objectives** outline the specific changes that need to be made to reach each goal.[2] Objectives should be SMART, i.e., Specific, Measurable, Accessible, Realistic, and Time-limited. The objectives should be able to answer the following questions: Who is the population being addressed? What is the specific change you desire? By when will the change be achieved? How much change is anticipated and in what direction should the change occur? How will change be measured? An example of a good objective is: 20% of students aged 13-17 who are exposed to the exercise training class intervention will be able to state five ways of exercising on a post-test by the end of the school year, as compared to pre-test measures. The goals and objectives of your project determine the rest of the plan. If your project involves comparing outcomes between groups of participants, the objectives could be stated as hypotheses that will lead to the quantitative method of statistical testing. If your project seeks to identify domains, or elements, of a problem, the objectives should specify what will be measured and how, and what qualitative methods will be used.

Strategies and activities provide the step-by-step road map. A new employee or volunteer should be able to discern who is doing what and when. This component of your plan specifies the design of the intervention, the people to be included, numbers involved, timeline, and persons responsible for implementing activities. The plans specified here will allow you to determine the resources needed. Use an intervention that has worked in other settings or try a new one, depending on what you uncover in your literature review. There is no need to "reinvent the wheel," especially if others have shown a specific intervention to be successful. If you have questions, call the authors; most will be delighted to discuss the particulars of their projects with you.

After the goals, objectives, strategies, and activities have been written, list the **resources** needed to accomplish each objective and corresponding task. This list should describe potential and existing sources of funding, supplies, facilities, people, and political allies. The availability of resources, or lack thereof, may limit the scope of your intervention.[2]

Identify **constraints**. You do not want to develop an entire intervention plan only to realize that you overlooked a key political opponent who can block your whole plan. You will probably be surprised by how many constraints you identify that are also listed as your resources.[2] When you list resources that are not immediately available, their absence becomes a constraint until they are developed. This applies also to political constraints. If you know of someone who may try to block your efforts, list that person or organization as a constraint until a strategy can be developed to bring that person around as an ally. To quote Dignan and Carr, "Neither resources nor constraints can be either utilized or affected unless they are first recognized, analyzed, and fully understood."[2]

Table 8.1 suggests one specific outline for an intervention plan that can be adapted to your program. If you decide to apply for funding from a governmental or private agency, your planning document contains a written record that you can shape into a proposal with little effort.[2]

You cannot completely plan your intervention unless you have also planned how to evaluate it. This implies that you have calculated or determined the sample size of the target population, designed process evaluation techniques, and determined the specific outcome measures to be used.

Implementing the Intervention

If you have carefully planned the implementation strategy, taking into account known obstacles, it will be easier to solve the unanticipated ones because you have already established group processes to deal with problems. When a change occurs in the plan, it will be helpful if you also change your planning document to reflect the change.

TABLE 8.1
Outline for Intervention Planning Document

I.   Introduction
    A.   Statement of the problem
    B.   Rationale for selecting specific at-risk subpopulation
    C.   Expected outcomes of the intervention

II. Literature Review
    A.   Previous successful interventions
    B.   Previous populations used

III. Goals, Objectives and Hypotheses
    A.   Overall program goals
    B.   Specific objectives for each goal
    C.   Hypotheses to be tested (if applicable)

IV. Methods
    A.   Subjects
    B.   Evaluation (study) design
    C.   Sample size
    D.   Intervention description
    E.   Measurable outcomes
    F.   Data management procedures
    G.   Analysis techniques

V.   Resources and constraints

    A.   Resources needed
    B.   Resources available
    C.   Constraints
    D.   Plan for overcoming constraints

VI. Implementation Plan
    A.   Detailed list of objectives
    B.   Activities and strategies, by objective
    B.   Timeline, by objective and activity

VII. Evaluation Plan

VIII. Budget

Dignan and Carr outline five phases of implementing an intervention.[2] The first phase is gaining acceptance for the program. If you have taken the steps to include the community in your planning process, as outlined throughout this book, the intervention plan will already be accepted by the community, the COPC team, and any other advisory groups with whom you are working.

In the second phase, review the planning document and make detailed lists of tasks necessary to accomplish each objective. Then, list the resources needed including money, people, time, and materials. Personnel is usually the highest cost item.[2] Regardless of whether personnel are paid or volunteer, each person assigned a task must be qualified to tackle the task or should be properly trained if necessary. Qualification criteria and training needs, therefore, should also be included in the plan.

You probably cannot sustain a longitudinal COPC effort that includes multiple projects over many years with grant money alone. And if you rely too heavily on grant money, your entire COPC effort may collapse when the grant money runs out. Alternative funding sources may include local fundraising activities or private and state grants. A sponsoring medical primary care practice or managed care organization may devote a yearly sum to COPC. The important part of raising money is to have a specific goal. If you fall short, do not implement the intervention piecemeal, but scale your entire plan back to match your resources.

The third phase, marketing your project, allows you to "sell" your plan to the community, to other health-related entities, to your specific subpopulation, and possibly to a funding agency. Marketing strategies need to be planned just like all other components of the COPC process. The plan should include the marketing goals, the specific information that is to be conveyed, a list of potential marketing strategies, activities and resources lists, and evaluation criteria to determine the extent to which your message is getting across. In COPC, potential strategies might include posters or fliers, free public service announcements on television and radio, visits to various civic groups, local health fairs, or producing a short film.

In the fourth phase, establish a mechanism for managing the implementation of the intervention (see Chapter 4). You will have to specify indicators to allow the COPC team to monitor progress, timeline, and cost.[2] This system of process evaluation using performance variables will help the team keep control of the implementation process. The data should be easy to collect. The fifth phase is the implementation of the intervention.

DESIGNING YOUR EVALUATION

The evaluation process is one of inquiry and, while a science in its own right, is not limited by strict rules.[2] The key is flexibility in approach. There is a practical trade-off between the feasibility of an evaluation and the rigor of project design.[3] Any intervention should be evaluated as rigorously as possible to determine its impact, but resources may limit the rigor. The purpose of the evaluation is to determine the effects of the intervention in your community, to provide useful feedback to the program planners, and in doing so, to assure credibility of the project to your team and community.[3] It will help you decide to continue the intervention as is, modify it, or discontinue it. Your evaluation does not have to be as rigorous as a formal research project, but the more rigorously you plan and evaluate your intervention, the better your chances are of showing the true impact of your project.

The evaluation is guided by the original program objectives.[4,5] It can assess both major aspects of the COPC process: the procedures and activities of the team (the process) and the effectiveness of the intervention (the outcome). Walker lists the following reasons for including evaluation as an integral part of COPC projects[1]:

▶ Evaluation is vital to the development of community-oriented primary care. It will help identify effective methods of improving health in your community.

▶ Evaluation is necessary for the most efficient use of resources.

▶ Evaluation is necessary to provide feedback.

▶ Evaluation is necessary to manage projects in progress.

▶ The process of evaluation may identify new areas and methods for future intervention.

▶ Evaluation is necessary to justify expenditures for research.

Since most health professionals practicing in community settings do not have expertise or experience designing evaluation methods, seeking technical assistance might be very beneficial. Scientific expertise can be found at universities and colleges, state and local health departments, some extension services and sometimes from community people with previous experience. Focus on practical issues of study questions, evaluation design, selecting measurable outcome variables, data collection and management techniques, and the approach to analysis. The earlier you involve technical consultants in the process, the better your outcome.

Process and Outcome Measures

Evaluations fall into two broad categories: process and outcome. In order to truly understand if your intervention has been successful at changing behavior (the outcome), you will first need to document whether or not the intervention occurred, how it occurred, and who was exposed to it. This is called process evaluation. Outcome data must be associated with program activities in order to explain any changes that occur in the measurements as a result of the intervention.[6] Changes in long-term outcomes (for example, reduction in births to teenagers), and short-term outcomes (knowledge, attitudes, and reported sexual behaviors) can only be attributed to the intervention if it took place, if it is clear who was exposed to it, and if it is understood how it was implemented. Process evaluation also enables you to make mid-course corrections when you have feedback that the intervention is not occurring as planned. Very often we mistakenly assume that the intervention was implemented as planned without any documentation of that fact, then later on we see that there were no outcome effects. The natural question asked in this situation is "Did the intervention occur as planned?" Only later do we hear horror stories that provide an explanation for the problem: the posters were still sitting in the district health officers' office, the radio station only played the spots between 2-4 am, bad weather prevented the training sessions from being held, and on and on. It would be more useful if that information were available during the intervention, so it could be corrected, rather than after the fact. Finally, a process evaluation can also help eliminate concerns that the changes were due to historical or external effects (called contamination) by documenting what other activities or environmental factors might have had a contributing effect to the changes in outcome measures.

As an example, process measures for a parenting class might include attendance records, documentation of the intended curriculum, facilitator logs documenting what was actually taught, and some feedback from the participants.

Outcome evaluation, on the other hand, measures change in the outcome indicators for the problem you are studying. These indicators can be focused at various levels of influence: individual, social network, community, structural or organizational, or policy. For example, if you are working on the problem of teen pregnancy, your community group may have decided that there are contributing problems at each level. At the policy level, the policy that allows pregnant or parenting teenage girls to become emancipated adults may be an incentive to getting pregnant. You may believe that lack of after-school activities contributes to the problem by giving teenagers too much unsupervised time. You may decide that the community attitude towards teen pregnancy is too lenient and permissive. Parents may believe they do not have skills to talk with their children about sex. Girls who are doing poorly in school and have low self-esteem may be at higher risk for pregnancy than those who are doing well and exhibit higher self-esteem. All of these contribute to your final outcome, the incidence rate of teen pregnancy. Each of these factors then becomes an indicator for the success of your intervention. They lead you to develop specific strategies and activities to overcome these problems in the same way they lead you to design an evaluation to measure any changes occurring at the various levels as influenced by your intervention.

Decisions about your evaluation design stem directly from the indicators you have selected to measure. Using the teen pregnancy indicators as an example, a complex evaluation design might emerge. Table 8.2 shows these multiple levels and provides examples of process and outcome evaluation measures that would accommodate all the indicators.

More measures and different types of measures enable you to have more confidence in your results, because the different types of measures will complement each other and confirm the results.

EVALUATION METHODS
Qualitative *and* quantitative methods of evaluation are used in most COPC projects. The type of evaluation you choose depends on the type of question you are asking.

TABLE 8.2

Designing an Evaluation for Multiple Levels of Analysis

Evaluation Levels	Process Evaluation Measures	Outcome Evaluation Measures
Policy Level: Change in policy emancipating pregnant teens	Document discussions leading to policy changes; media attention; lobbying of political leaders; vote on policy	Actual change in policy
Structural/Organizational Level: Increase number of after-school activities	Document discussions about after-school activities; document line-item budget allocation of after-school activities	Count number of after-school activities pre- and post-intervention
Community Level: Change in community members' attitudes about teen pregnancy	Document media/public relations campaign about community attitudes to teen pregnancy	Survey of community members pre- and post-intervention to determine changes in attitudes
Social Network Level: Improvement in parent communication skills	Document parent communication classes; document parents in attendance; document types of skills addressed	Survey of parents attending classes pre- and post-intervention to determine changes in skills (actual or perceived)
Individual Level (Impact): Decrease numbers of girls who are doing poorly in school; improvement in girls' self-esteem	Document special attention to girls doing poorly; document self-esteem classes or curriculum; document numbers of girls in attendance	Count numbers of girls doing poorly pre- and post-intervention; survey of self-esteem measures in girls pre- and post-intervention
Individual Level (Outcome): Decrease frequency of teen pregnancy	Document proportion of teen girls receiving multifaceted intervention program	Measure rate of births to teen girls

Qualitative methods such as focus group discussions, in-depth interviews, and participant observation are increasingly being used in evaluation research in order to enhance information obtained from more traditional quantitative methods. Qualitative methods can be used to:

▶ Collect information to develop a quantitative instrument, such as a survey.

▶ Understand the range of possible responses to an issue.

▶ Better understand the results of a survey.

▶ Understand "how and why" instead of "what and how many."

▶ Develop hypotheses for future testing.

Qualitative methods are not simple, cheap, subjective, or time saving. If you are asking: "How many people..." then you need to use a quantitative method. If you are asking: "How did the people interpret the message..." then you might be better off with a qualitative method. Qualitative methods bring depth and context to a topic; you use them to learn about the range of available information.

Quantitative methods are used when you want a numerical analysis of outcomes, a statistical model to predict outcomes, or hypothesis tests.

QUALITATIVE METHODS
Evaluation Design
Three commonly used qualitative methods are focus groups, in-depth interviews, and observation.

Focus Groups
The focus group discussion technique is also addressed in Chapter 5. Information is obtained from a group of six to 10 people simultaneously. The interaction among the participants encourages more discussion and often reveals different types of information than an in-depth interview of one person. A focus group discussion tends to reveal "social norms," information that people are comfortable discussing with other members of the group.

There is the misperception that focus group discussions are a quick and easy research tool; this could not be further from the truth. Focus group discussions require a skilled moderator and a note-taker. These people must be trained in probing and following leads (see in-depth interview, below). A focus group discussion uses a focus group guide: a list of five to ten topics that the moderator must cover during the focus group, along with some sample questions and probes. The guide normally begins with a "warm up" question that may or may not be part of the primary focus group discussion topic; its purpose is to get everyone in the group talking about a topic that is easy for them to talk about. The entire discussion can last from one to one-and-a-half hours. Before any discussion takes place, it is useful to establish "ground rules" for the discussion. These may include items such as talking one at a time, or the need for confidentiality and anonymity, no right or wrong answers, etc. Making sure that everyone expresses his or her opinion in a manner that encourages interaction and participation can be a challenge. Focus group discussions are most often tape-recorded. It's often a good idea to have two tape recorders going, one started a few minutes before the other, so that no conversation is lost when the first side of the tape runs out and it is time to turn it over.

In-depth Interviews

In-depth interviewing is a compromise between unstructured and semi-structured interviewing techniques. An in-depth interview is basically a one-on-one conversation that uses an interview guide as the basis for discussion. The interview begins with specific initial questions. The interviewer can then use other skills including probing and following leads to elicit more in-depth information. The specific questions ensure that all informants are asked the same questions in the same manner. Probing and following leads will allow the interviewer to get more in-depth responses to the initial questions. The purpose of the semi-structured format is to control the context in which the information is given, so that many respondents' answers can be compared.

In general, there are three main types of questions used in in-depth interviews: descriptive, structural, and contrastive. Descriptive questions ask the informant to describe an experience, a place, or an event. "I have never attended a parenting class. Could you describe it for me?" is an example. Structural questions are aimed at discovering how informants organize their knowledge; they are, therefore, best for uncovering categories or domains. For example, you might ask informants to tell you the different kinds of activities that are offered in the community for youths; once they provide you with a list you might ask them to organize the items on the list into categories. Contrastive questions attempt to understand exactly what an informant means by a term he or she uses. A contrastive question might ask the informant to clarify the differences between two types of activities that have been mentioned. For example, we might take the responses to the above question about youth activities and ask the informant to identify the differences between two or more activities.

In-depth interviewing requires the skills of probing and following leads, and may include other techniques such as free-listing, rank-ordering, and the development of taxonomies and scales, all of which are explained in detail elsewhere.[7,8] Probing is the skill of stimulating a respondent to produce more information on a particular topic without injecting the interviewer's ideas into the discussion. The most common type of probe is to repeat back to the respondent what he has said and ask for more information. Another way to probe is to nod affirmatively after being given information, encouraging the respondent to continue along the same vein.

Following leads is a way for the interviewer to pick up on the responses of the informant, even if the information given is slightly off the topic at hand. Informants will rarely give all the information you request the first time a question is asked but may provide information after having thought about the topic for awhile.

Observation
There are two kinds of observation: participatory and structured. Participatory observation implies that you participate as you observe. For example, to find out if a group of parents has learned new communication skills, you might attend an interactive workshop of parents with their children; you might go along as a parent with your child and participate, but the real purpose for your participation is to observe what the other parents are doing. Structured observation implies that you have a structured form on which you are entering data. For example, you might observe people exercising, and at every 60-second interval you might write down what exercises the persons who you have selected to observe are doing.

Observation can be intrusive and may initially affect the behavior of observed participants. For this reason, allow enough time for the observed participants to forget that they are being observed and to get back into their normal behavior pattern. This usually can take from a few minutes to one hour, depending on the type of activity being observed, and how obvious it is that you are conducting an observation.

It is more difficult than it appears to get consistent results from different observers. For this reason, observers should be very clear about the purpose of their observation and exactly what they are observing. The best kind of observation is video recording, because the individual observer is not the only decision-maker about the content of the observation. If you choose this route, have participants sign an informed consent.

Sampling
Qualitative sampling is purposeful. For example, if you are interested in learning grocery shoppers' impressions about a nutrition display, go to a grocery store and interview a certain number of people after they have seen the display. Despite its purposeful nature, qualitative sampling is systematic and often includes random selection.

A sampling frame is usually devised that defines the different characteristics of persons (male/female, ethnic group, ill/healthy), or geographic locations (urban/suburban) that you think will make a difference in the answers you might get, or which constitute your intervention area. The rule of thumb is to select three to five persons (or hold three to five focus groups) for each characteristic you think is important to include. Table 8.3 shows how the number of characteristics you include increases your sample number exponentially. For four characteristics (gender, ethnicity, age and geographic location) you would need 24 groups, each having 3-5 people, for a total of 72 (at three respondents per cell), or 120 (at five respondents per cell), who would be recruited to participate in your qualitative method. This means that the numbers of people interviewed or the numbers of focus groups held can get quite large.

Data Management
Transcribing Data
Analyzing the data from a focus group or an in-depth interview is a multi-step and lengthy process. First the tape recordings must be transcribed. A

TABLE 8.3
Typical Sampling Frame for Qualitative Methods
(Showing minimum of three participants per cell)

GENDER (female, male)	ETHNICITY (Hispanic, Native American, Caucasian)	AGE (25-49, 50-65)	GEOGRAPHIC LOCATION (urban, suburban)
3	3	3	3
			3
		3	3
			3
	3	3	3
			3
		3	3
			3
	3	3	3
			3
		3	3
			3
3	3	3	3
			3
		3	3
			3
	3	3	3
			3
		3	3
			3
	3	3	3
			3
		3	3
			3

one-hour focus group discussion or in-depth interview can take four hours or more to transcribe. After the transcriptionist has typed the transcript it is often necessary to review the transcription while listening to the tape recording to catch all the errors made in the transcription. This can take another four hours.

Once the data are transcribed, they must be coded. Developing a coding format for qualitative data is a lengthy process because it involves reading the data, not just creating a framework based on the questions asked, as when quantitative methods are being used.

Coding Data

If you will be using a computer to analyze your data, each piece of information you collect will need to be named for input into a database. For both qualitative and quantitative data, develop a coding format or codebook, which explains how each variable is coded. Qualitative data codes evolve from the combination of the interview guide and what transpires during the focus groups, interview or observation. You will need to read the transcribed data to arrive at a full set of codes. Coding formats are organized into family trees; the "grandparents" are the cover term for all the codes that fall underneath it (see Figure 8.1). They are the major subheadings of the data. Codes at each subsequent level ("parents") ("children") are equivalent categories. For most qualitative data you probably won't need to go further than three generations of codes. Codes are not interpretive; rather, we create codes that organize the data as they are reported. For example, if the question were, "Could you please give me a list of fruits that are being sold in this store today?", FRUIT would be the "grandparent" code (1.00). Under that; if the respondent told you that there were categories of fruits, e.g., those that are picked off a tree, those that are picked off a bush, and those that grow in the ground; the "parent" codes would be TREE (1.01), BUSH (1.02), and GROUND (1.03). If the respondent went further to describe characteristics about fruits from trees (1.01), the resulting lists of fruits in this category might be further broken down into the "children" coded headings FRUIT WITH EDIBLE SKIN (1.01.01), FRUIT WITH INEDIBLE SKIN (1.01.02), and so forth.

After you have created your coding tree, read over the transcript and mark the codes (usually in the right hand margin) that apply to each piece of the transcript. Often a piece of text will include information for several codes. Once your transcripts have been coded, they can be entered into a computer program which will compile and summarize the data, or you can do this by hand. The first step of compiling the data by either method would be to gather all the coded data together in groups. For example, all statements about "fruit with edible skins" would be put together, and reviewed. There would probably be a great deal of similarities in respondents' statements, but there would likely be some differences. These similarities and differences can then be summarized.

FIGURE 8.1: Qualitative Evaluation Coding Tree

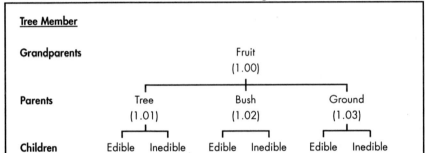

Tree Member			
Grandparents		Fruit (1.00)	
Parents	Tree (1.01)	Bush (1.02)	Ground (1.03)
Children	Edible (1.01.01) Inedible (1.01.02)	Edible (1.02.01) Inedible (1.02.02)	Edible (1.03.01) Inedible (1.03.02)

Analysis
If you are analyzing qualitative data by hand, take the coded data, compile them, summarize them, and analyze them to answer the questions you have posed. A good way of organizing qualitative data is to put them in a matrix. Once you have summarized the data, there are several kinds of analyses that you can undertake.

Content Analysis
Content analysis is basically a descriptive summary of the total data set. To examine all the press coverage on your intervention topic, to see whether it had received primarily positive or negative coverage, list all newspaper, TV, and radio stories on your matrix. Summarize the content of each, perhaps looking for accuracy, positive or negative slant, referral to the program, etc. Then you would be able to determine, overall, the range of press coverage; you would also be able to count the numbers of different pieces of information and calculate the proportion that fit into

each of your categories of concern. This is one time when you can use both qualitative and quantitative methods on the same data set.

Creating Domains
A domain is a category that contains four elements: a cover term, two or more included terms, a single semantic relationship, and a boundary. Cover terms are names for categories of items. "Fruit" is a cover term for a category of foods that grow off the ground. "Included terms" are items that belong to the category; for example, "apple" and "banana". All domains have a single semantic relationship, which means that they are linked together. "Apple" *is a kind of* "fruit". The words "*is a kind of*" denote the semantic relationship. All domains have boundaries; i.e., items which cannot be included in the domain. For example, a cucumber is not a fruit, but rather a vegetable (a different domain). Earlier we used an example of fruit sold at a market to discuss the coding of data. Using the same example, FRUIT is a category of foods that are not vegetables, meat, dairy products or grains. The domain of "Fruit" can be further divided in many ways: by how they grow, by their skin, by their color, etc. When you ask an informant to give you this kind of information you are learning about how people categorize items.

Context or Meaning
Most of the reason we use qualitative methods is to discover the context or meaning of a topic in more depth than can be provided by quantitative methods. For example, we may want to know what people think about teen pregnancy but we also might like to understand how they think about teen pregnancy in relationship to other problems in the community, such as alcoholism or gang violence. It may be that these topics are interrelated in a way that would not be uncovered by asking about each topic separately.

QUANTITATIVE METHODS
The ultimate goal in evaluating the intervention is to judge whether or not it has been successful in meeting your goals for changing a community health problem. This assessment is the culmination of all your planning efforts and reflects all the decisions that have been made in developing your project.[2] The actual quantitative assessment usually involves comparing

numerical "indicators of success" of the intervention between a population or group that received the intervention and one that didn't. Indicators you choose to measure depend on the question being asked, the problem being addressed, and on what level of that problem the intervention is focused. The specific statistical analysis that will be performed is determined by the type of indicators you choose and the design of the evaluation.

Many good resources exist on the specifics of epidemiological and statistical measurements, designs and formulae.[7-13] In this section we discuss how to approach a quantitative analysis. As in qualitative methods, the question being asked defines the type of variables to be measured, the (study) design of the evaluation, and the statistical measures needed. Consult a statistician to help you plan data collection and analysis if you are not experienced in statistical analysis.

When information about a community is collected through primary or secondary data sources, the data can be shaped into a computerized database. This shaping process, what we call data management, includes coding the indicator variables, entering them into the database from your questionnaire or survey, verifying that the values for each variable are correct, and editing the data where necessary.

In statistical terms, your analysis will be comparing an indicator variable in one group to the same variable in another group, and your statistical test will tell you the probability of getting the observed difference by chance if in reality there is no difference (the p-value). Assuming no bias existed in the way you chose your groups or measured them, you may infer that your intervention probably caused the observed difference.

The analysis can be performed using a logical stepwise approach. After the database has been constructed, become familiar with your data. Describe each variable thoroughly, which can usually be done simply in database management, spreadsheet, or statistical software programs. Calculate the mean and median, the range, standard deviation, percentiles, and any descriptive statistics (proportions, percentages, ratios and rates) that are appropriate. If your analysis is descriptive, you can stop after this step.

Most quantitative analyses, though, involve comparing at least one variable between two groups. First, perform a univariate analysis by comparing the predictor, or independent, variables one at a time to the outcome, or dependent, variables. For example, we recently performed a survey looking at the use of herbal remedies in an elderly clinic population.[14]

The principal outcome variable was the proportion of study participants who used herbs, and the principal question was whether or not there was a difference between Hispanic and Anglo herb use. Other extraneous factors we thought might be important in explaining the variation in herbal use were income, education, age, and gender. During the univariate step we compared each of the predictor variables in turn to the main outcome variable, herbal use. We found that each predictor variable was associated with a significant difference in the proportion of our sample who used herbs. In order to account for those differences while still comparing Hispanic and Anglo herb use, we used multivariate statistical techniques.

Multivariate analysis can be used to test your main predictor, or independent, variable against your outcome, or dependent, variable while controlling for other extraneous variables. This procedure mathematically equalizes the extraneous variables between the groups being compared and allows you to interpret the association between the dependent and independent variables, given that the extraneous variables were equally distributed between the groups being tested. In the herb study, we performed a multivariate analysis comparing herb use between Hispanics and Anglos controlling for the extraneous variables of income, age, education, and gender. We found that a significantly higher percentage of Hispanics used herbs than Anglos even when the extraneous variables were controlled, indicating a true ethnic difference in herb use.

Types of Data (Measurement Scales)

Once you have decided on the specific level of health problem to study, the target sub-population, and the general aims of your intervention, it's time to think about what kind of information you will need to evaluate your intervention. It's useful to think about this information in terms of sets of observations, on which you want to collect information. For example, if your aim is to improve blood lipid levels using an exercise intervention, you will at least want to determine before and after levels of the serum total cholesterol, HDL, LDL and triglycerides. These measurements (in total) constitute a set of outcome observations you will want to track for each participant in your intervention program.

The variables you decide to measure need to be organized in a logical manner that makes most sense to you in terms of desired outcome. The way you organize and classify these variables will determine the statistical procedure you will use to evaluate your intervention. Quantitative variables can be organized into *continuous* or *discrete* variables.[9] Continuous variables implies unbroken and uninterrupted, and means that between any two numbers for that variable there is another number that bridges the gap and makes the scale unbroken. Thus we consider continuous variables to be measuring a possible interval of values. For example, a person's diastolic blood pressure could be 90.5, or 90.05, or 90.005 mm Hg. Between any of these numbers it is theoretically possible to have another value for the measurement. Discrete variables, on the other hand, have gaps between them — a broken scale. Discrete variables are "count" data, i.e.; they can be counted in whole numbers. Therefore, proportions, often used in COPC projects, are discrete variables. They usually represent information that can be counted or different levels of one variable that can be counted. For example, it may be more meaningful to divide diastolic blood pressure levels into risk categories rather than represent it as a continuous variable, and count the number who have pressures in each category, e.g., those with pressures less than 80, 81-90, 91-100 mm Hg, etc. If discrete variables are ordered to reflect the magnitude of the categories, they are called ordinal variables because they can be put in order. If the discrete variables you collect have no magnitude, and are merely identifiers, they are referred to as nominal variables because they are identified by name.[12] Examples include gender, ethnicity, zip code, participant identification number and so on (see Table 8.4).

TABLE 8.4
Discrete and Continuous Variables

Variables	Discrete	Discrete Type	Continuous
BP, systolic	1 if < 140 mm. 2 if ≥ 140 and < 160 3 if ≥ 160	Ordinal	BP, mm Hg.
Cholesterol	1 if < 200 Cholesterol mg/dl 2 if ≥ 200	Ordinal	mg/dl
Gender	1 if male; 2 if female	Nominal	Not applicable

The type of measurement scale you use to classify your data will determine the type of statistical test you will use to analyze your results. Different types of data use different tests. Continuous data can use a student's t-test for separate groups or a paired t-test if two measurements on the same individual over time are being compared. Discrete data use a chi-squared test. The details of these and many other statistical tests can be provided by a technical consultant or statistics texts.[9,10,13]

Evaluation Designs

COPC projects are usually concerned with changing some risky health behavior in an identified population. In order to measure change in any indicator variable, the measurement has to be performed at least twice, before and after the intervention. This type of evaluation design can be considered an experimental design, also called a clinical trial or intervention study,[2,11,12,15] because it involves manipulating the study group in some way (the intervention) and then determining if there was any effect. Many writings on COPC have suggested using the classic designs of epidemiology, but we have found that the ones used most are this type of experimental method. Case control or cohort (study) designs are observational methods, usually used to determine risk factors for a given disease[12]; they are not used much in COPC projects because they do not involve interventions; they are not experimental.[2]

A big decision is whether or not to use a comparison group. At a minimum, plan to measure your group before and after the intervention. But without a comparison group that did not receive the intervention, you don't know if the change in behavior you observed would have occurred without the intervention over the period of follow-up. Including a comparison group takes more effort in monitoring and costs more because the number of participants is larger. On the other hand, it is scientifically much more sound and provides a basis for comparison.

Practical considerations also enter into the decision. Sometimes you cannot prevent a comparison group from being exposed to an intervention, especially if your activities have been widely advertised or if the intervention is a community-wide program. If a local comparison group will be "contaminated" (from a scientific standpoint), you may be able to choose a similar comparison group from a nearby community. The following evaluation designs are the ones most likely to be used in COPC projects.

Before-After Intervention, Comparison Group Design (Figure 8.2)
This design involves a pre-intervention assessment of the comparison group and the intervention group, and a post-intervention assessment using the same groups and measurements. An important assumption for this design is that the comparison and intervention groups are as similar as possible and represent the same at-risk subpopulation. After deciding on the criteria for inclusion of subjects, use random allocation to divide people into two groups (see Appendix 8.1). Random allocation is used to ensure that each qualified participant has an equal chance of being in the comparison or intervention group, thus theoretically avoiding bias, or systematic error, in the group selection process. You may recognize this design as a randomized, controlled clinical trial (Figure 8.2).[2,11,12,15] After allocation to the comparison groups the indicator outcomes are measured similarly in both groups. Any changes in the indicator outcome variables can be attributed to the effect of the intervention. If for some reason you cannot divide the eligible population into two groups, you can still perform a before-after design using a comparison group from another community (Before-After Intervention, Comparison Group from Different Community Populations, Figure 8.2).

Before-After Intervention, No Comparison Group
When you cannot use a comparison group, usually because of restricted resources or unavailability of a similar but separate eligible population, you can use the same participant group and measure their outcome variables before and after the intervention. If you decide on this design, you are implicitly making the assumption that there would be no change in the outcome variables over time if there were no intervention. This design is not as technically sound as those using a comparison group.

After-Intervention Only, Comparison Group
When pre-intervention assessment is not possible, you may use a post-intervention-only assessment, but in this case, it is essential to use a comparison group. You should never plan to just measure the groups on whom you intervened once the intervention is complete.

Selection of a comparison group for this design uses the same assumption as for the designs discussed above, that the two groups are similar and come from the same subpopulation. Randomization is the best method for allocating subjects to the two groups. This is especially impor-

FIGURE 8.2: Quantitative Evaluation Designs

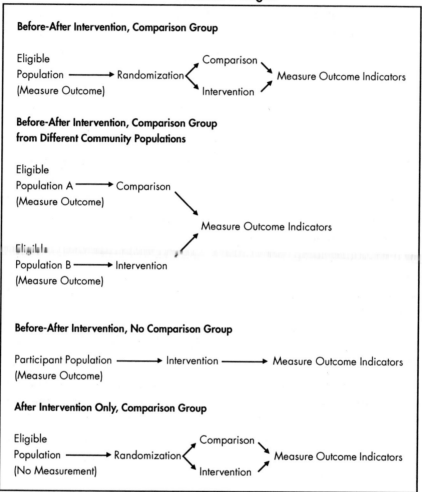

tant in this design because you will not be able to compare the two groups before the intervention.

Without a pre-intervention assessment or a comparison group, you are left with one measurement on your participant group, a situation that makes it impossible to assess the impact of your intervention.

Sample Size: How Many Subjects?

In order to plan the intervention and the evaluation, you must know how many subjects you will need in each study group. During the planning phases this will allow you to better estimate needed resources. To determine sample size you will need to know, or estimate:

▶ How big the impact of the intervention will need to be in order for it to be important to you. This is the clinically important difference in your outcome variable you expect to detect.

▶ The direction of the estimated differences. If the outcome variable for the intervention group could logically turn out to be either larger or smaller than for the comparison group, use a "two-tailed" procedure. (Ask yourself if there is any possibility that the change could go in the unexpected direction, e.g., sometimes people who exercise gain weight.) If you can specify the direction of the difference beyond a reasonable doubt, then and only then, use the "one-tailed" procedure.

▶ Type I and Type II statistical error rates you are willing to accept. A Type I error occurs when you detect an intervention effect that your statistical test says is significantly different from the comparison group when, in reality, there is no difference. This is similar to a false positive test. The probability of a Type I error is also called the alpha level or level of significance. It is the probability that the observed significant difference is due to chance alone, or random error. The level of significance is usually specified by convention to be 0.05. A Type II error occurs when you fail to detect a significant intervention effect when in reality there is one. This is similar to a false negative test.

▶ Statistical power. Specify the chance that a Type II error will not occur. That is, it is the probability of being able to detect a significant difference of a specified size if that difference actually does exist. The probability of a Type II error is also called the beta error. Power is equal to one minus beta (1-beta=power). Therefore, Type II error is the probability that you *will not* detect a difference if one exists, and power is the probability that you *will* detect a difference if one exists. Power is usually specified to be 0.80 or 0.90.

▶ If the outcome variable is continuous you will also need an estimate of the standard deviation, or variance. To a large extent, choosing a sample size involves a trade-off between the logistics of including more people and the desire to be able to detect fairly small differences between the two groups.

The graphs in Appendix 8.2 can be used to determine approximate sample size for differences between proportions by specifying these parameters.

As an example, suppose your community wants to institute a smoking cessation program. The outcome will be a comparison of the proportion of people who quit smoking in a non-intervention, or comparison, group with the proportion of people who quit smoking in an intervention group. The intervention is a behavioral program that takes six months to complete. From a baseline survey from the state health department you determine that 24% of your population is likely to smoke. Assume that after looking at results obtained by other people, you estimate that approximately 10% of people in the intervention group will quit smoking during the six-month period. However, you are not willing to rule out the chance that the proportion of people quitting smoking in the intervention group will be smaller than the proportion of people quitting in the comparison group, so you will specify a two-tailed test. You would like to have at least an 80% chance of detecting that difference if it exists (i.e., statistical power of at least 80%). Assume that the statistical test will be done at the 5% level of significance (Type I error). That is, there is a 5% probability of finding an effect by chance alone even if there is no effect. In order to detect that size of difference with 80% power you will need approximately 250 people in each group. If you want the power to be 70%, then you will need about 200 people in each group, and you will need about 300 people in each group if you want the power to be 90%. In general, increasing power increases sample size requirements. As you can see from Appendix 8.2, the relationship is not linear. As you get closer to 100% power the necessary sample sizes increase rapidly. As the size of the effect you want to be able to detect decreases, the sample size increases. The relationship is an inverse square root relationship. That is, if you quadruple the sample size you will be able to detect a difference that is 1/2 of the difference you would be able to detect with the smaller sample size. If you multiply the sample size by nine you will be able to detect a difference that is 1/3 of the difference you would be able to detect with the smaller sample size.

Data Management

The major steps of data management usually involve:

a. Coding data.

If you are constructing a computer database, you will need to create abbreviated code names that make sense to you. For example, the code name for whether or not a person is a smoker may be SMOKE or SMK and will be coded as a 0 if the participant does not smoke or 1 if he or she is a smoker. Our practice is to code a "yes" response as a "1" and a "no" response as a "0". The quantity a person smokes may be SMKQNTY and will be entered as a numeric value representing the number of cigarettes smoked daily.

b. Data entry.

When writing a survey or questionnaire, it is useful to put the name of the variable by the coded response so that data entry is easier. This should be done in such a way that it does not confuse the respondent or make the questionnaire difficult to understand. The data can be input easier if the question and the various potential responses are on the left side of the page and the variable code name and specific response to the question is on the right side of the page. This allows the person entering data to keep track of the variables and to enter data quickly using the vertical list of variables on the right hand portion of the page. (See Chapter 6, Example 6.1)

Once your questionnaires are completed and before analyzing the data, you need to verify that the responses are coded correctly and that there are no errors of data input. Review each questionnaire to see that each question has a response, that the proper response is recorded and that it is transcribed correctly on the data entry portions of the questionnaire. Some people prefer to have separate data entry forms and some incorporate the data entry portion into their original questionnaires. Still others design questionnaires on laptop computers so that the respondents answer the questions using the computer and the data are entered directly into the computer. Which method you use depends on your resources and computer capability.

c. Validating and editing data

After the data have been entered into a computer database, you need to check for errors of data entry. For smaller data sets, print out a list of responses and manually check them against the questionnaires. For larger data sets, where manual checks are not feasible, you must rely on computer maneuvers to validate your data. You can calculate the range of the variables and inspect them to see if they are reasonable or if there are "nonsense" values that lie outside the expected ranges. Another procedure is to perform the data entry twice and use software that matches each response and prints out the ones that are different.

d. Plans for analyzing the data.

Are you going to use statistical procedures for data description, estimation, or hypothesis testing? Do you just want to describe what you have in your sample or do you want to generalize the results from this sample to a larger population? If you want to generalize, are you doing estimation or hypothesis testing? Estimation procedures are designed to calculate the numerical value of variables from the data. For example, how much was the mean cholesterol value changed by the intervention? Did the intervention result in a statistically significant lowering of the mean cholesterol value? Both estimation and hypothesis testing take sampling variation into account. Hypothesis testing helps make the decision of whether or not there is a statistically significant difference between variables.

USING THE INFORMATION
TO IMPROVE YOUR PROGRAM (FEEDBACK LOOP)

You evaluate process and outcome to learn through a feedback mechanism whether you need to change something you are doing. First, evaluating the process tells you if you need to change the current program. If the intervention or evaluation is not being performed as planned, you can change it now. For example, the authors were involved in a project evaluating a curriculum for sixth graders on pregnancy prevention. The curriculum was being taught by the students' regular teachers, who had received training in the new curriculum. By evaluating the lessons, we saw that some of the teachers were not implementing the curriculum as planned. They changed some aspects of the curriculum and were teaching what they thought was correct, which was different from the planned curriculum. The problem was corrected by providing those teachers with more individualized training.

Outcome evaluation suggests new or revised interventions in the future. When you have successfully evaluated an intervention, you get feedback on whether it changed something about a health problem. Sometimes you can determine that one subpopulation was affected more than another, which implies that subsequent interventions can be focused on those specific subpopulations. For example, evaluating a teen pregnancy intervention showed that girls who get pregnant have lower self-esteem. This information helped the team focus their next intervention on those girls. The intervention was also changed to one that was designed to raise self-esteem, rather than focus on sexual and pregnancy prevention behavior.

REFERENCES

1. Walker RB. Evaluating impact in COPC. In: Nutting PA, ed. *Community-Oriented Primary Care: From Principle to Practice*. US Department of Health and Human Services, Health Resources and Services Administration; 1987;339-340.
2. Dignan MB, Carr PA. *Program Planning for Health Education and Health Promotion*. Philadelphia, Penn: Lea and Febiger; 1987.
3. Nutting PA, ed. *Community-Oriented Primary Care: From Principle to Practice*. Washington, DC: US Dept of Health and Human Services, Health Resources and Services Administration; 1987; 336.
4. Overall NA, Williamson J, eds. *Community-Oriented Primary Care in Action: A Practice Manual for Primary Care Settings*. University of California at Berkeley, 1987, p. 55.
5. Roher JE. Planning for community-oriented health systems. Washington, DC: APHA; 1996.
6. Windsor R, Baranowshki T, Cutter G. *Evaluation of Health Promotion, Health Education, and Disease Prevention Programs*. 2nd ed. Mountain View, Calif: Mayfield; 1994.
7. Bernard HR. *Research Methods in Anthropology, Qualitative and Quantitative Approaches*. 2nd ed. Thousand Oaks, Calif: Sage Publications; 1994.
8. Spradley J. *The Ethnographic Interview*. Austin, Tex: Holt, Rinehart, and Winston; 1979.
9. Saunders BD, Trapp RG. *Basic and Clinical Biostatistics*. East Norwalk, Conn: Appleton and Lange; 1990.
10. Kuzma JW. *Basic Statistics for the Health Sciences*. Palo Alto, Calif: Mayfield Publishing Company; 1984.
11. Fletcher RH, Fletcher SW, Wagner EH. *Clinical Epidemiology: The Essentials*. 2nd ed. Baltimore, Md: Williams and Wilkins; 1988.
12. Hennekens CH, Baring JE. *Epidemiology in Medicine*. London, England: Little Brown; 1990.
13. Shott S. *Statistics for Health Professionals*. Philadelphia, Penn: WB Saunders; 1990.
14. Rhyne et al. The interface of phytotherapy and allopathic medicine in an elderly clinic population. *Alternative Therapies*. 1997;3:101-2.
15. Hulley SB, Cummings SR. *Designing Clinical Research: An Epidemiologic Approach*. Baltimore, Md: Williams and Wilkins; 1988.

CHAPTER 9

Incorporating
COPC Into Primary Care

David Garr
Margaret Kelsey

ABSTRACT

The newest definition of primary care challenges clinicians to expand their roles to serve the community. Though extensively trained in individual care, clinicians will need to learn the population skills covered in this book to succeed in COPC. Training in epidemiology is not enough because COPC is based on population-based measurement and planning in an ongoing process of community collaboration, problem identification, intervention, evaluation, and feedback—with more emphasis on disease prevention and health promotion. Clinicians need not undertake a major community-based project all at once, but can shift to COPC in phases, concentrating first on subpopulations within their practices and gradually broadening their services to include entire communities. The recent shift toward managed care organizations (MCOs) will advance COPC because some MCOs provide more preventive care than do traditional fee-for-service practices. In addition, many MCOs already have the multidisciplinary work force, outreach programs, and centralized structure necessary for COPC initiatives. New compensation and benefit packages are incentives for practicing COPC. Utilizing teamwork and computerized records, a practice can become more successful and save both time and money through COPC.

INTRODUCTION

Times are changing. An Institute of Medicine (IOM) report in 1978 defined primary care as accessible, acceptable, comprehensive, coordinated, continuous over time, and accountable.[1] In 1996, the IOM defined primary care as "the provision of integrated, accessible health care services by clinicians who are accountable for addressing a large majority of personal health care needs, developing a sustained partnership with patients, and practicing in the context of family and community."[2]

The new definition poses a challenge for primary care providers; to have them expand their role from providing services to individuals who seek care to assuming a responsibility for their practice population as a whole and, whenever possible, to assist with health care for the larger community in which the practice resides.[3] Managed care organizations (MCOs) are focusing more on populations, and will probably do so more in the future. They are becoming more concerned with preventing disease in their enrolled populations as a mechanism to optimize the cost of caring for people with illness. As managed care evolves, this is a good time for primary care providers to work with MCOs to address the needs of populations and to begin to change the incentive structure so that providers have incentives for changing behaviors in populations and MCOs have incentives for addressing health problems in communities. COPC implies a significant role for primary care providers in partnering with others to care for populations and communities.[4]

THE SHIFT FROM PRIMARY CARE
TO COMMUNITY-ORIENTED PRIMARY CARE

How realistic is it to expect clinicians to change from the traditional primary care model to one that incorporates the COPC approach? The answer will depend in large part on the commitment of the clinicians and the additional effort required. As shown in Table 9.1, the COPC transformation occurs when a primary care practice introduces a more expansive view of the role of the clinicians and the practice in serving the community.[5]

The medical provider is trained extensively in the clinical skills necessary to care for individual patients, but usually lacks the population skills required to practice COPC. Early writings described COPC as a combination of epidemiologic skills with primary care skills. However, the authors in this book have found that, while classic epidemiologic skills certainly deal with disease patterns in populations, they are not enough to convert the average clinician into a COPC practitioner. The classic study designs used in epidemiology are rarely used in COPC (see Chapter 8 for a discussion of evaluation designs). The skills described in this book are more appropriate for the COPC practitioner. The two sets of skills overlap but COPC uses more of the community organizing, quasi-experimental and qualitative evaluation skills; thus, in Table 9.1 the methods are described as "epidemiologic-type" skills. COPC differs from epidemiology and is special because of its use of population-based measurement and planning in an *ongoing process* of problem identification, intervention, evaluation and feedback. It is conducted as a collaboration among clinicians and other community members working as a team.

TABLE 9.1
Shifting from Primary Care to COPC

Clinical Domain	Primary Care	+ Community Approach = COPC
Focus on Unit of Care	Patients seen as individuals	+ Patients seen as members of a population
	Emphasis on active users	Emphasis on active users and non-users
Method to Assess Health Needs	Patient-oriented Clinical skills	+ Population-oriented Epidemiologic-type skills
Planning	Primarily concerned with utilization by active users	+ Health needs of the community served
Use of Work Force	Medical specialties and ancillary staff	+ Multiple community and health professional participants possessing a range of skills
Intervention	Individualized patient education and treatment	+ Community outreach prevention programs
Assessment of Outcomes	Health of the individual patient	+ Health status of an identified population

Adapted from Overall NA, Williamson J, eds. *Community-Oriented Primary Care in Action: A Practice Manual for Primary Care Settings.* University of California at Berkeley, 1987, p 4.

Interventions in primary care involve individual patient education and treatment. In the past, the clinical focus has been mostly on treatment and monitoring of disease states; in COPC, the focus shifts not only to populations, but much more to disease prevention and health promotion.

MOVING TO COPC IN PHASES

The shift to a COPC approach can proceed in phases. A clinician does not have to jump directly into a community-based project. He or she might begin with a population of practice users, then expand to a population of users and their families, then move to a user and non-user population that resides in the practice service area, then finally to a larger geographic area community-based population. For example, a practice interested in the care of diabetic patients might first identify all the diabetic patients in the practice and the demographic characteristics of this population.[6] A meeting with a group of diabetic patients could be organized to solicit ways in which the practice could be more effective in meeting their needs. This patient group could assist in the creation of new programs and services within the practice or help identify services already available in the community. A practice could sponsor exercise and health education classes for diabetic patients and monitor a variety of outcome parameters, e.g., blood glucose control, use of medications, hospitalization rate.

To continue with the same example, a higher level of COPC activity could focus on both the users and non-users of a clinical practice who live in the community. Clinicians, staff, and patients might join with other health care practices or patient groups in the community to broaden the participation and interest in the new services for diabetics. These practices and clinicians might be affiliated with the same MCO or integrated health care delivery system. The result could be the development of a comprehensive program in which many people work together to increase the range and quality of health care services for diabetics in the community.

Population-based initiatives can be successful if there is sufficient interest and commitment from a variety of community members and other health professionals in developing community intervention programs to meet identified needs. It may be difficult for a small practice that is just beginning COPC to lead such a large effort. It might be more appropriate at this level of activity to partner with others and form a COPC team with wide representation. This takes the onus off the practice as the principal leader of the COPC process.

HOW MANAGED CARE CAN ADVANCE THE PRACTICE OF COPC

The transition from fee-for-service care to managed care has been gradual until the past few years, when the pace has rapidly accelerated. This expansion of managed care has significant implications for primary care in general and for community-oriented care in particular. Studies have shown that some MCOs, especially health maintenance organizations (HMOs), cover more preventive care services and patients receive more preventive care than in traditional fee-for-service practices.[7-11] Clinicians providing care to HMO-insured patients are more willing to provide preventive services since such services are covered and encouraged by the HMO plan.

Another type of MCO which is becoming more common is the integrated delivery system (IDS). An IDS is a vertically integrated health care system which facilitates the coordination of patient care across multiple disciplines of the health care continuum. For clinicians interested in initiating a COPC effort, the multidisciplinary work force needed for a COPC initiative is often already in place in an IDS as are pathways of communication among members of the IDS workforce. For COPC purposes, the IDS is "vastly superior to the previous health care delivery paradigm, characterized by independent physician and stand alone hospitals focused on the provision of acute care."[12]

The introduction of performance measures, like the Health Plan Employer Data and Information Set (HEDIS), has increased the attention MCOs pay to the health of the populations they are serving.[13,14] Access by the public to data comparing the performance of MCOs has increased the prevalence of outreach programs by MCOs to their patients as they seek to improve the health profile of their patient population.[15,16] In coming years, it is likely that community-oriented care will emerge as one of the benefits touted prominently by MCOs. It will behoove them to also become involved in COPC-type processes for their enrollee population and the communities they serve.

COPC LEADERSHIP

Not all primary care is provided by physicians in their offices. Nurse practitioners, physician assistants, and advanced practice nurses are involved with increasing frequency. Likewise, not all COPC initiatives require clinicians or primary care practices as the principal leaders. Rather, what is needed is a commitment to collaborate among a diverse group of people with one or more members designated as the leaders.

The centralized administrative structure of MCOs can help provide the coordination and leadership to address the needs of groups of people within the health care system. For example, an effort undertaken by an MCO to improve the care provided to people with diabetes could use the quality improvement staff to work with diabetics, informing them about programs and services available to them, as well as providing guidance to clinicians about the newest standards for diabetes care. Thus, clinicians, patients, staff, and others in the community could all work together with the quality improvement personnel to form a COPC team that would implement and evaluate the community-oriented program for diabetics (see Chapter 3 on COPC teams).

ADVANTAGES AND OBSTACLES

Incentives

The process of adopting a population-based approach to delivering clinical services can give rise to a level of involvement and visibility of the practice's providers and staff in the surrounding community that had not previously existed. These outreach efforts combined with greater practice visibility can result in an increase in the prominence and popularity of the practice. The incentives, or lack of incentives, for practicing COPC have not changed in the last 15 years.[16,17] As mentioned, economic and organizational barriers have limited participation of clinicians and patients in the COPC process, but these barriers are now coming down.[18,19] The resource-based relative value scale (RBRVS) compensates clinicians for providing education and counseling services to their patients. In addition, the benefits packages provided by many insurers now pay for an expansive range of preventive services. These recent developments, combined with the recommendations by the US Preventive Services Task Force,[20] are providing incentives for clinicians to adopt a community-oriented approach to care. In addition, MCOs are examining the health profiles of patients in clinicians' practices. Those whose results match or exceed the targeted levels are receiving financial rewards. For example, in some systems practices whose immunization rates for children exceed a certain threshold receive an additional financial reimbursement.

Time

One of the first concerns cited by clinicians is that they do not have time to undertake more activities. While this concern is valid, a community-oriented approach might actually relieve some of the demands placed on clinicians, especially where capitation plays a large role in one's practice. Using the example of diabetic patients, preventive care through the community-oriented approach can decrease the frequency of complications, . With the increased prevalence of managed care and capitation, decreased morbidity translates into a reduced cost of care with greater cost savings for the insurer and fewer office visits.

Teamwork

The goal of any COPC process can be reached without placing undue burden on any individual if people work together to attain the goals of the program (see Chapter 3). A key to successful initiatives is a multidisciplinary team that works efficiently to divide the responsibilities for planning, implementing, and evaluating the project. An added benefit of the team approach is the rapport, trust, and enthusiasm that can develop. It helps to have an administrative structure and a specific person identified as the coordinator of the process who oversees the details of daily tasks.

Medical schools and residency training programs are looking for clinical sites where students and residents can work in communities and acquire experience in community-oriented care. These learners can become members of the team and provide a useful service to community-oriented efforts.

Accessing Information

Comprehensive, affordable, user-friendly computerized medical records systems can assist with the provision of population-based health care. Research has shown that computer-generated reminders for patients and physicians can increase the use of preventive services.[21-27] Computer systems permit easier access to information about patients in a clinical practice. Practices without computer systems must rely on manual methods for retrieving population information. It is anticipated that computerized medical records will eventually replace paper medical records, facilitating the incorporation of community-oriented approaches into primary care. MCOs and hospitals often have computerized databases that can be used to access information. They may also be able to help construct computerized monitoring systems that will help you evaluate the effects of the intervention.

CONCLUSION

The future design of the US health care system has generated considerable debate in recent years. The definition of primary care has been changed to include community. And, the community-oriented primary care model has been cited as one that can be useful when planning the health care system of the future.[18,19] The COPC approach, because of its population-based emphasis, is well suited for meeting the health needs of the American people. This opportunity is reflected in the interest that has emerged in building a closer relationship between medicine and public health.[28] The shift from primary care to COPC requires appreciating the population and community approach and learning new skills that have usually not been taught in traditional medical education, but are contained in this volume.

The health care system in the United States depends on the provision of excellent primary care. Yet, the limitations imposed by the traditional 1:1 approach used in the provision of primary care services have resulted in unrealized potential for the provision of high quality preventive and curative health care services. Historically, clinicians have relied on the motivation and initiative of individuals to acquire the health care services they needed. COPC provides an opportunity for primary care practitioners to expand their range of services and to work closely with their communities to better meet the needs of the people they serve. Incorporating COPC into primary health care has the potential to make a major contribution in reshaping health care in the United States.

REFERENCES

1. National Academy of Sciences, Institute of Medicine. *A Manpower Policy for Primary Health Care*. Washington, DC: National Academy Press; 1978.
2. Donaldson MS, Yordy KD, Lohr KN, Vanselow NA, eds. *Primary Care: America's Health in a New Era*. Washington, DC: National Academy Press; 1996.
3. Greenlick MR. Educating physicians for population-based clinical practice. *JAMA*.1992; 267:1645-48.
4. Mullan F. Community-oriented primary care: an agenda for the 80's. *NEJM*.1982; 307:1076-8.
5. Garr D, Rhyne R, Kukulka G. Incorporating a community-oriented approach into primary care. *Am Fam Phys*. 1993; 47:1698-1701.
6. Nutting PA, Garr DR. *Community-Oriented Primary Care*. Home Study Self-Assessment Program. Kansas City, Mo; 1989. American Academy of Family Physicians. Working Paper 124.

7. Diehr PK, et al. Utilization: ambulatory and hospital. In: Richardson WC, ed. *The Seattle Prepaid Health Care Project: Comparison of Health Services Delivery.* National Technical Information Service; 1976. PB267488-SET.

8. Luft HS. *Health Maintenance Organizations: Dimensions of Performance.* New York, NY: John Wiley; 1981.

9. Miller RH, Luft HS. Managed care plan performance since 1980: a literature analysis. *JAMA.* 1994; 271(pt 19):1512-9.

10. Schauffler HH, Rodriguez T. Availability and utilization of health promotion programs and satisfaction with health plan. *Med Care.* 1994; 32(pt 12):1182-96.

11. Shortell SM, Gillies RR, Anderson DA, Erikson KM, Mitchell JB. *Remaking Health Care in America.* San Francisco, Calif: Jossey-Bass; 1996.

12. Sennett C. Introduction to HEDIS - The health plan employer data & information set. *JCOM.* 1996; 3:59-61.

13. Thompson RS. What have HMOs learned about clinical prevention services? An examination of the experience at Group Health Cooperative of Puget Sound. *The Milbank Quarterly.*1996; 4:469-509.

14. Baker EL, et al. Health reform and the health of the public: forging community health partnerships. *JAMA.*1994; 272:1276-82.

15. Rundall TG, Shaffler HH. Health promotion and disease prevention in integrated delivery systems: the role of market forces. *Am J Prev Med.* 1997; 13 (pt 4):244-50.

16. O'Connor PJ. Is community-oriented primary care a viable concept in actual practice? An opposing view. *J Fam Pract.* 1989; 28:206-208.

17. Rogers DE. Community-oriented primary care. *JAMA.*1982; 248:1622-25.

18. Wright RA. Community-oriented primary care: the cornerstone of health care reform. *JAMA.*1993; 269:2544-47.

19. O'Connor PJ. Community-oriented primary care in a brave new world. *Arch Fam Med.*1994; 3:493-94.

20. US Preventive Services Task Force. *Guide to clinical preventive services.* 2nd ed. Baltimore, Md: Williams & Wilkins, 1996.

21. McDonald CJ, Hui SL, Smith DM, Tierney WM, Cohen SJ, Weinberger M, et al. Reminders to physicians from an introspective computer medical record: A two-year randomized trial. *Ann Int Med.*1984; 100:130-138.

22. Tierney WM, Hui SL, McDonald CJ. Delayed feedback of physician performance versus immediate reminders to perform preventive care: events on physician compliance. *Medical Care.* 1986; 24:659-666.

23. Tape TG, Givner N, Wigton RS, Seelig CB, Patil K, Campbell JR. Process in ambulatory care: a controlled clinical trial of computerized records. *Symposium on Computer Applications in Medical Care.* 1988; 749-752.

24. Harris RP, O'Malley MS, Fletcher S, Knight BP. Prompting physicians for preventive procedures: a five-year study of manual and computer reminders. *Am J Prev Med.* 1990; 6:145-152.

25. Ornstein SM, Garr DR, Jenkins RG, Rust PF, Arnon A. Computer-generated physician and patient reminders: tools to improve population adherence to selected preventive services. *J Fam Pract.* 1991; 32:82-90.

26. McPhee SJ, Bird JA, Fordham D, Rodnick JE, Osborn EH. Promoting cancer prevention activities by primary care physicians: results of a randomized, controlled trial. *JAMA.* 1991; 266:538-544.

27. McDowell I, Newell C, Rosser W. Computerized reminders to encourage cervical screening in family practice. *J Fam Pract.* 1989; 28:420-424.

28. Lasker RD and the Committee on Medicine and Public Health. *Medicine & Public Health: The Power of Collaboration.* New York: The New York Academy of Medicine; 1997.

CHAPTER 10

Education and Training in Community-Oriented Primary Care

Suzanne Cashman

Ron Anderson

Hugh Fulmer

ABSTRACT

Educators responsible for COPC programs can draw on the successful experiences of the clinical sciences in producing practitioners skilled in one-on-one patient care. Many of the same principles apply: the teaching staff must accept responsibility for the health of the patient—in this case, the community; students must have role models; the full range of COPC activities must be covered; students must learn coordination skills in order to work as a team as well as skills in evaluating the results of interventions; they need adequate time to contribute to a community partnership; and they must participate actively. Providing clinical services in a community is not learning COPC; specific times must be set aside for COPC activities. Specific competencies needed in COPC are discussed. The authors outline a model COPC curriculum and discuss the effective use of cluster committees to introduce trainees to the process. Barriers to COPC training still exist, including needs for institutional vision, faculty expertise, dedicated curriculum time, trust within the community, and a supportive external environment. However, the continued growth of managed care, with its emphasis on health promotion and disease prevention, will exert pressure for change.

INTRODUCTION

The study of COPC can excite health care professionals. It is action-oriented, broad in scope, and grounded in the community. It connects practitioners to communities, forging partnerships that can improve a community's health and quality of life. By applying COPC principles, health care professionals can achieve their goal of improving health status.[1,2] Unlike one-on-one clinical care, COPC focuses on improving the health of groups of people. COPC practitioners, therefore, need to apply principles of population health sciences and work as a team as they confront the broad dimensions of health as well as illness.[3]

Many students in the health professions begin their education open to the idea of taking responsibility for a community's health. Unless they learn the skills of COPC, however, they probably will limit their focus to individual patients. If health care practitioners are to care for a community's health, they need to learn how. Otherwise, a lack of confidence and competence will keep them in their offices, disengaged from the pertinent community issues. Professional role models can help students develop their sense of responsibility for a community's health by teaching them the relevant skills.

PARALLELS TO EDUCATION AND
TRAINING IN THE CLINICAL SCIENCES

For many years, students in American programs have received exemplary education in the clinical sciences. US academic health centers and their teaching hospitals are regarded as world leaders. Lessons from these successes can be learned for COPC. Parallels between the scientific practice of medicine, nursing, or other clinical disciplines and the scientific practice of COPC provide a helpful framework for teachers and students. As shown in Table 10.1, the clinician's approach and actions *vis a vis* the individual patient parallel the approach and actions *vis a vis* a community. The essence in COPC is that the community is the "patient" and the practitioner expends the same effort to understand, work with, diagnose, and apply a treatment plan.[4,5]

Lessons learned from teaching the clinical sciences include, first, the basic necessity of having the proper environment: the requisite facilities, staff, and support. *Facilities* might include primary care practices, community teaching hospitals, transportation, and computers and accompanying

TABLE 10.1
Parallel Between Clinical Care and COPC

Clinical Care	Step	COPC
Who is the patient?	1	Define and characterize the community
Engage the patient; initiate practitioner-patient relationship	2	Involve the community; initiate the community-professional partnership
Differential diagnosis	3	Conduct a community diagnosis; rank issues in priority order
Treatment	4	Develop and implement an intervention
Follow-up; is the patient improving?	5	Monitor and evaluate

software for data analysis. *Staff* refers to the array of personnel of various levels and backgrounds necessary in any primary care and public health practice. *Support* is represented by the availability of funds to cover operating expenses for the full range of COPC activities.

Second, lessons from the clinical sciences suggest that several *elements* are necessary for teaching the process of COPC. These include responsibility, role models, activities, coordination, evaluation, time, and participation. *Responsibility* refers to the teaching staff's clear definition of their own and the field faculty's responsibility for a community's health. The health care facility must be in accord. (Indeed, ideally, the parameters of staff responsibility would be developed in accordance with the health care facility's mission.) *Role models* captures the importance of students having competent, inspiring mentors. Just as clinicians in training learn to provide high quality clinical care through clinical *activities* on a teaching service, students of COPC need to be trained in an environment where the range of skills described in this book are being applied.

Coordination is taught and modeled for students in clinical services so that efficient, effective teamwork is assured. Similarly, the student joins the COPC team that collaborates responsibly and efficiently in carrying out each of the five steps of COPC. In the clinical setting, careful monitoring and follow-up of patients is an ongoing task that students learn and practice. In the community, students of COPC learn to apply methods of *evaluation* to monitor the effectiveness of interventions.

Time is often understood implicitly to be a necessary ingredient of the educational experience; it is being made explicit here because it is critical, and sometimes ignored. Just as clinical students need adequate time to be exposed to the total process of patient care, COPC requires adequate time in the curriculum to contribute to building a partnership with a community, to understanding its range of health problems as well as the resources available to it, to exploring the methods available for improving health, to developing and applying an intervention plan, and to monitoring outcomes. The mistake often made is assuming a student learns COPC by providing clinical services in a community setting. Time must be set aside, separate from providing clinical care, for students to become involved in COPC activities. Given the demands on students' and residents' time, however, unless taught as a focus of a fellowship, it is unlikely that COPC activities in which any one student engages will be more than a slice of the full model of COPC. This increases the need to have faculty who are practicing COPC so that students can piggyback onto COPC activities.

Finally, *participation* is essential. Students of clinical care have the opportunity to participate with the patient in learning to cultivate the practitioner-patient relationship; similarly, students of COPC must have opportunities to participate actively and meaningfully in caring for and with the community.

MODELS OF TRAINING IN THE CLINICAL SCIENCES

A significant component of training in COPC is applied experience. Just as clinical skills cannot be learned properly without the opportunity to apply them in a learning situation, community health skills cannot be learned exclusively in the classroom and need to be applied in real communities, in relation to real issues.[6,7] As explained in Chapter 6, one very practical, pragmatic way to begin institutionalizing this application is for the student of COPC to examine a practice and plot the patient population on a map. This process produces a powerful visual that prompts interest in understanding the larger demographic profile.[8]

For physicians, education and training consist of medical school, residency, fellowship, and continuing education. Although the educational avenues for becoming a nurse are more varied, advancement traditionally has come through enrolling in certificate programs or pursuing degrees; continuing education is mandatory.[9] Many other health care practitioners are required to complete continuing education and can pursue advanced degrees. COPC should be a factor in each of the stages of health care practitioners' education and training.

Students in medical school and undergraduate health professions programs should be introduced to COPC through a combination of classroom instruction in population and community health sciences and practical experience in the community.[10] This reflects the model used to teach clinical skills.[11,12,13] The basic sciences that form the theoretical and academic basis for COPC practice consist of 1) social/behavioral sciences, 2) epidemiology, 3) biostatistics, 4) leadership and administration, 5) environmental health, and 6) disease prevention/health promotion. Although many of these topics are already taught in undergraduate health professions training schools, they are not taught from the perspective of COPC. They form the core of graduate programs in public health, but their curricular expression is not yet oriented toward COPC. Nevertheless, they represent an important base for developing the following COPC skills: community health assessment; fostering and leading collective action; collecting, analyzing, and interpreting data; developing and managing the operation and financing of a health program; and developing methods to prevent disease.

COPC can be introduced by classroom instruction. However, this instruction needs to be supplemented with experiential practice with the community as the classroom. The trainee may be assigned to a community, where he or she functions as part of a team, working to express the definition of public health, i.e., "organized community efforts aimed at the prevention of disease and promotion of health. It links many disciplines and rests upon the scientific core of epidemiology."[14] Through regular clerkships or rotations, students begin to relate to a community.[15,16] It is important that the experience be structured as part of a faculty group's ongoing relationship to a community. Students are under intense time pressure, and their situation is transient. They need to participate without bearing the entire weight of a community health effort.

Faculty skilled in—and committed to—COPC help ensure that experiential work provides an opportunity for students to apply and polish skills and knowledge, as well as to develop critical attitudes. Attitudes are central to the success of COPC education and training.[12,17] One essential attitude that forms the basis of COPC is feeling a shared responsibility for the community in its entirety, i.e., those individuals who do, as well as those who do not, use health services. This is a crucial and fundamental difference between the practice of high quality primary care and high quality primary care that is community oriented and responsive to the community.

If not fully integrated into a practice's *modus operandi*, COPC efforts run the risk of being just another ancillary service or specialty performed by members of a health care team. In those cases, what people would have pass for COPC is really just a health promotion/disease prevention project that does not express the depth and breadth of work that is COPC.

ACADEMIC HEALTH CENTERS AND COPC

COPC challenges the very foundations of academic health centers (AHCs) and what has caused them to be successful institutions.[18] But market forces and political reforms mean that AHCs must reshape themselves in order to succeed in this continually evolving managed care environment, whose emphasis is on ambulatory care. Prevention needs to be incorporated at all levels and in all specialties. The community needs to be seen as a source of opportunity rather than a chaotic drain. Given the increasing diversity of society and the recognition that care must be provided within the patients' value and belief system, AHCs will need to view patients and communities as partners in the healing process.[19,20] Finally, publicly supported universities have a responsibility to give back to the community. This obligation might be partially met through providing support for 1) further development of COPC curriculum materials, 2) faculty development in COPC, and 3) outcomes research that focuses on the results of developing COPC practice sites.

Structures currently in place in AHCs can be restructured to support COPC by:

▶ Building a COPC curriculum in existing population-based academic departments such as preventive medicine, community medicine, family medicine, and social and behavioral medicine.

▶ Collaborating with schools of public health, the Centers for Disease Control and Prevention, and state departments of public health to provide population-based training and linkages to non-hospital based training sites.

▶ Linking with health care systems, managed care organizations, and health departments to access population-based practices.

Although ideally the knowledge, skills, and attitudes needed to practice COPC would be taught from the start of any health professional's education they can be taught at any juncture. Formal, post-graduate residency and residency-type training programs can include both classroom sessions and hands-on experiences. While training in COPC is particularly pertinent to post-graduate programs in preventive medicine, family medicine, and community/public health nursing, it can be incorporated readily into any of the primary care specialties. (Indeed, in 1993, the federal Public Health Service made COPC a priority for funding its primary care training grant programs. Unfortunately, the focus was the four step, truncated version of COPC, rather than the five step approach that this book advocates.) In addition, COPC-related instruction can be incorporated into all specialty training programs; this type of instruction is critical if health care practitioners are to contribute to ensuring that the health care system is responsive to the community.[21] If the commitment to this type of practice exists, developing the didactic modules is straightforward and uncomplicated. Potentially more problematic is ensuring that the practices in which the trainees are placed are COPC practices that will help initiate neophyte professionals.

Given that it is never too late to learn the theory and practice of COPC, the core principles can also be taught as part of continuing professional education. This can be accomplished through intensive multi-day certificate programs, as well as longer-term, less intense training. The key always is to develop practice or practice-like experiences for trainees. Working with communities is new and intimidating for many health care professionals; it is important that mentors guide them in their initiation into community health work.

COMPETENCIES

With the Institute of Medicine's 1988 report, *The Future of Public Health*, which called for a recommitment to leadership in public health, professional associations, academic departments, training programs, and the federal government initiated or revisited efforts to articulate competencies for their education and training programs.[22] Defined as what people should be able to do, rather than what they should know,[23] competencies needed to practice COPC reflect the six areas of basic science, i.e., social/behavioral sciences, epidemiology, biostatistics, leadership and administration, environmental health, and disease prevention/health promotion.

Competency specification provides a central locus for trainers, educators, mentors, and role models to make it possible to conduct an inventory of their current capabilities and qualifications. In addition, the process provides an avenue for designing/redesigning and supporting new faculty development programs.

Competencies for the practice of COPC reflect many of the areas of expertise that have been identified by the American College of Preventive Medicine,[24] the Public Health Faculty/Agency Forum,[25] the Pew Health Professions Commission,[26] and the Public Health Functions Project of the federal Public Health Service.[27] In the Pew Commission's initial report, members stated that their Agenda for Action indicated that for change to occur, a significant number of health care educators (e.g., physicians, nurses, and allied health professionals) must accept the values and beliefs inherent in the recommended changes and be willing to translate these values into curriculum changes. Additionally, they reported that "the nation must have practitioners with expanded abilities and new attitudes to meet society's evolving health care needs." Members specified those abilities and attitudes through defining seventeen competencies that health care professionals for the year 2005 should master. The first two competencies, "care for the community's health" and "expand access to effective care," relate centrally to COPC.

Members of the Public Health Functions Project took a slightly different approach from the Pew Commission's. Rather than specify competencies for individual practitioners, they specified competencies that facilities or agencies need in order to provide 10 essential public health services:[27]

1. Monitor health status to identify community health problems.

2. Diagnose and investigate health problems and health hazards in the community.

3. Inform, educate, and empower people about health issues.

4. Mobilize community partnerships to identify and solve problems.

5. Develop policies and plans that support individual and community health efforts.

6. Enforce laws and regulations that protect health and ensure safety.

7. Link people to needed personal health services and ensure the provision of health care when otherwise unavailable.

8. Assure a competent public health and personal health care workforce.

9. Evaluate effectiveness, accessibility, and quality of personal and population-based health services.

10. Research for new insights and innovative solutions to health problems.

Within each of these essential services, members of the Project have specified competencies that encompass skills in communication, policy and development/program planning, cultural issues, financial planning and management, and basic public health sciences. Programs that educate and train health care professionals to merge clinical care with public health will find these competencies a useful starting (or revising) point for developing/renewing the program. The breadth and depth of the competencies render them cogent for undergraduate, graduate, fellowship, and continuing education, as well as formal faculty development programs.

THE COPC CURRICULUM

At the heart of any curriculum in COPC is the notion that the practitioner team and facility assume a responsibility for the health of a defined population, a community, and engage in activities aimed at improving the health and therefore the quality of life of that community. The key difference in teaching clinical skills and skills needed for public health rests in the concept of the denominator. Given COPC's integration of clinical medicine and public health, training in COPC ensures that clinicians develop the requisite knowledge, attitudes, and skills for providing individual care as well as community care.

The COPC curriculum aims to train practitioners to engage in a type of practice that goes beyond strictly a high quality primary care practice. It trains practitioners for change at two levels: one, the individual practitioner who merges clinical medicine and public health, and two, the institution, organization, or agency that develops linkages with community members to ensure the growth of a valid and viable community-professional partnership.[28] Training in COPC stresses the importance of the contribution that local citizens can make to improving the health of a community; the health care agenda is no longer mainly the purview of the professional.

The didactic component of education in COPC can be structured to introduce technical skills within the topical areas of the five steps of COPC. As with any curriculum, learning goals need to be specified, appropriate readings listed, and teaching activities planned and evaluated. We suggest an outline below, incorporating the six areas of basic science mentioned earlier, but the emphasis is on application. They can be expanded or distilled. Given the skill level and background of trainees, the learning goals can emphasize either the theoretical or the practical. We recommend a mix of lecture/discussion, role play, and small group activities.

    I.   Introduction to Community-Responsive Systems of Care

          A.   Historical context and COPC; need to merge medicine and public health; concept of community-responsive systems of care; Medicine/Public Health Initiative;

Preventive Medicine and COPC; Blueprint for a Healthy Community; amalgamating health care business and principles of community health

B. Learning Goals

1. Understand definitions of public health, community, primary care, community-responsive care, community-oriented primary care, and healthy communities.

2. Understand the schism between medicine and public health and how COPC merges the two.

3. Understand and be able to identify indicators of health and the factors that contribute to the health of a community.

4. Understand the concept of a community health improvement process and the various national and federal tools for applying the process.

5. Explore the developing nexus between the business of health care and care for communities.

II. Defining and Characterizing the Community

A. Rudiments of demography, concept of community and populations, systems analysis, secondary and primary data sources

B. Learning Goals

1. Understand the distinction between community and population and how this affects community definition; become familiar with how community has been viewed historically; introduce John Gardner's ingredients of community[29] and the National Civic League's civil society.[30]

2. Consider basic epidemiologic factors in the definition and characterization of community;

know available data sources that describe communities.

3. Be able to identify and characterize the multiple communities to which a health care delivery system might relate, e.g., geographic, employee groups, capitated members, etc.

4. Understand relationship between defining community and ability to develop and implement successful programs.

5. Become acquainted with the way(s) official health agencies view community and how they relate to each other.

III. Involving the Community

A. Introduction to community organizing, theories of social change, group process, coalition development

B. Learning Goals

1. Consider theories of empowerment and be able to apply them in organizational settings; understand the connection between empowerment and health.

2. Understand the theory and concepts that underlie specific approaches to community organizing.

3. Learn ways that health care has been used as a basis for organizing communities and implications for providers and health care systems.

4. Discuss obstacles and supports for implementing community-responsive care.

5. Understand the components of organizational analysis.

6. Introduce a model for framing and analyzing issues.

IV. Community Diagnosis

A. Applied epidemiology; short feedback loop; causation; risk concepts; mapping assets and deficits; surveillance; environmental health

B. Learning Goals

1. Learn the definitions, strategies, and uses of epidemiology.

2. Understand the epidemiologic concept of cause; become knowledgeable about methods of determining and describing disease causation, including multiple causation.

3. Understand the concept of populations at risk, individual risk, relative risk, and attributable risk.

4. Be able to use basic methods of surveillance of acute and chronic disease incidence, prevalence, and distribution, and understand trends over time.

5. Know the tools available to conduct an environmental assessment and be able to apply them.

6. Be able to identify the major and potentially hidden problems and strengths of a community.

7. Understand the approach and uses of the Health Employer Data and Information Set (HEDIS), small area variation, and preventable hospitalizations in developing a community assessment.

8. Know the likely data sources and types of information available for community assessment.

V. Intervention Design and Implementation

A. Sociobehavioral sciences; program administration and organization; financial risk; connection to evaluation

B. Learning Goals

1. Be able to identify the determinants of a selected problem and focus on those determinants that are amenable to intervention.

2. Explore concept of financial risk and its relationship to the organization and delivery of a health promotion/disease prevention project.

3. Be able to specify the objectives of an intervention in measurable terms; understand the relationship between designing the intervention and designing the evaluation.

4. Consider multiple complementary levels and points at which the intervention can be implemented.

5. Understand the importance of identifying and coordinating the intervention with pre-existing pertinent programs.

6. Explore the concept of team; learn how interdisciplinary teams can be structured and how they function.

VI. Monitoring and Evaluation

A. Sociobehavioral sciences; management information; data analysis; evaluation methodologies

B. Learning Goals

1. Understand evaluation design and the importance of incorporating it into program planning. This includes qualitative and

quantitative methods, classic epidemiologic study designs and quasi-experimental designs.

2. Determine appropriate context, process and outcome measures; relate these to changes in health status in specific populations.

3. Be able to develop an evaluation design of appropriate rigor; consider characteristics of the intervention, available resources, and purpose of evaluation.

4. Understand the emergence of Hospital Community Benefits Standards/Guidelines as an evaluative standard for hospitals with applications to other organized systems of care delivery.

5. Explore the issue of balancing the savings of lives with the savings of money.

6. Be able to use Healthy Communities/Healthy People 2000 in setting appropriate objectives.

As already noted, the skills needed to practice COPC effectively cannot be learned exclusively in the classroom. In COPC, the community becomes a classroom of a different sort. Trainees who are expected to learn and apply COPC in practice sites must have dedicated time—apart from clinical practice—to apply the principles of COPC. We cannot stress too strongly that *simply practicing in a community-based setting and working on a health promotion project is not equivalent to learning and practicing COPC in a community*. The belief that a health promotion project based at a community health site constitutes COPC does a disservice by limiting it severely and ignoring the process that is COPC.

The practicum experiences must be sufficiently complete that, through them, practitioners understand that COPC is a way of practicing; it is looking continually at defined populations or communities and working with them to identify and address health problems. Understanding the process is critical for understanding ways in which professionals can develop partnerships with communities to improve health. In developing COPC education and training programs, it is important to know whether trainees are being placed at sites that are already practicing COPC, or whether they are at sites that would like to become COPC sites.

The differences are critical for the amount of leadership that the trainee will need to assume. When at a site that is committed to and skilled in COPC, trainees are in the familiar cocoon of training where everyone involved is working to develop a similar path toward the same goal. When placed at a site that is not yet practicing COPC, the trainee may need to engage with COPC faculty in education and training of other staff so that they understand and support the changes that are being initiated. This can be accomplished through several avenues, from developing an ongoing faculty development program (that may include trainees), to sending faculty to short certificate courses in COPC.

THE CLUSTER COMMITTEE

The cluster committee is an educational and catalytic activity conceived of and developed by the first residency and fellowship in preventive medicine and COPC in the country.[31,32] It is a very effective means both to advance COPC at a site that is already practicing in a community-responsive, denominator-sensitive way, as well as at a site that desires eventually to incorporate those attributes. The cluster committee process initiates a trainee's development of a unique set of competencies in community-related and leadership skills that merge medicine and public health (see Table 10.2). Simultaneously, the process is a vehicle for establishing linkages among the community, its public health sites, experts in public health, clinicians, and others training in the COPC model.

The cluster committee is designed to meet the following objectives:

▶ Initiate the trainee into the steps and processes of COPC.

▶ Educate community residents, health and human service agency practitioners, academicians, and local clinicians (site staff) about the COPC process.

▶ Provide assistance to the trainee by serving as a clinical, political, and technical resource.

TABLE 10.2
COPC Competencies Taught Through the Cluster Committee Process

1. Generic
   a. Order priorities according to a demonstrable systematic rationale
   b. Identify the decision-making process within an organization/agency and its points of influence
   c. Identify and obtain needed multidisciplinary skills to address a health issue

2. Communication and teaching skills
   a. Contribute to organizing and developing a multidisciplinary team
   b. Function effectively as a team member
   c. Able to facilitate a meeting
   d. Able to teach according to principles of adult learning
   e. Skilled in written communications
   f. Communicate in a clear and effective manner findings and rationale for selected interventions

3. Community-related skills
   a. Able to orient and work appropriately in a historical and organizational context
   b. Skilled in identifying and understanding multiple dimensions of the community
   c. Able to work with communities to identify and set priorities on community health problems
   d. Able to work with communities to plan and implement health interventions
   e. Able to contribute to organizing community groups and helping the community participate in activities that support community health programs
   f. Participate in community coalitions

4. Epidemiology/biostatistics
   a. Apply community-based epidemiology
   b. Presentation of epidemiologic data

5. Data evaluation skills
   a. Able to obtain and analyze primary and secondary data
   b. Able to monitor/evaluate/modify a health care intervention

6. Administrative
   a. Set goals and objectives for a given health issue
   b. Design an implementation plan to address goals and objectives
   c. Design an evaluation/quality assessment plan based on measurable criteria

7. Leadership skills
   a. Able to function as a change agent in promoting a site's advancement relative to COPC principles
   b. Demonstrate ability to identify conflict and negotiate effectively
   c. Able to take a lead role in improving a community's health and quality of life
   d. Able to take a lead role in using and applying new federal/national/state health planning tools

8. Cultural skills
   a. Interact sensitively, effectively, and professionally with persons from diverse cultural, socioeconomic, educational, and professional backgrounds
   b. Identify the role of cultural, social, and behavioral factors in determining disease, disease prevention, health-promoting behavior, and medical service organization and delivery
   c. Develop and adapt approaches to problems that take into account cultural differences

▶ Develop the leadership skills of the trainee for bringing about change.

▶ Encourage the development of relationships within the community that foster health promotion and disease prevention, and as such, begin the process of coalition building.

▶ Bring together the perspectives of community members, clinicians, academics, and public health practitioners regarding community health and focus on improving the health and quality of life within the community.

The cluster committee consists of four "subcommunities:"

▶ Staff of the community-based site where the trainee is placed.

▶ Community members.

▶ Representatives of academic institutions, community service organizations, and public governmental agencies.

▶ Other COPC trainees and program faculty.

Acting as a facilitator, the trainee leads the cluster committee in discussing one step of COPC at each of five meetings held at approximately one-month intervals. It is important for the trainee as well as the cluster committee members to understand that this series is an initial introduction. No one is actually carrying out each step of COPC to completion and using the meeting time to report his or her work. Rather, people who have a stake in a community's health participate in a structured format to learn about and discuss the process and steps of COPC, hear one another's views, and begin a planning process. The trainee's primary faculty mentor attends all meetings and leads debriefings; a field faculty member, usually based at the site, would also attend the cluster committee meetings and debriefings.

Cluster committee meetings are designed to follow the steps of COPC. A meeting may include 15-50 or more people and generally lasts for one and a half to two hours. The first meeting includes a definition of COPC, an outline of the process, and a sense of how a COPC practice might look as it cares for both numerator and denominator populations; then the first step of COPC, characterizing and describing the community, is discussed; the trainee might present demographic descriptors that he or she has obtained from census or town profile data. This presentation draws on many of the activities outlined and discussed in Chapter 6 and may serve as a basis for members to respond from their own experience or data. Application of basic mapping techniques that give a visual presentation of the community's geography as well as residence of patients seen at the site can provide a powerful tool for discussion.

At the second meeting, attendees brainstorm approaches to community organizing and strive to identify subgroups of the denominator that have not yet become involved. Many of the group process techniques discussed in Chapter 5 can be useful as a focus, particularly as the trainee is modeling the partnership development process that is fundamental to COPC. Specific outreach efforts may be identified, with participants volunteering to carry out certain efforts as a means to making the cluster committee as inclusive as possible.

The third meeting is spent laying the groundwork for a community diagnosis. Attendees identify community assets and resources and begin to articulate the health problems and issues of concern. Again, maps are effective visual aids. Demographic and secondary data that list major health problems of the community are also useful, along with people's impressions of major health problems. A nominal group technique (see Chapter 5) may be used to rank problems.

At the fourth and fifth meetings, members draft the parameters of a potential intervention to improve health, present disease parameters, and identify indicators of success for data gathering aimed at monitoring and evaluation. See Chapter 8 for a discussion of approaches to developing an intervention and a means to evaluate and monitor it.

At sites where the COPC approach might have been practiced for several years and several cluster committee series may have been held, subsequent meetings may take the form of revisiting and refining data for each of the steps. Alternatively, members may have evolved into a COPC team with which the trainee can work on specific health promotion/disease prevention programs. As in any community-based activity, while the overall plan and objectives for the cluster committee meetings and for the intervention itself can and should be specified, the details of how they are carried out are often shaped by the process.

Any program that uses the cluster committee approach to teach COPC should have all trainees attend the cluster committee series of their colleagues. Just as it is important for students to see and work with a variety of patients, it is important for students and practitioners of COPC to see and understand the complexities of a variety of communities. By attending and helping debrief others' cluster committee meetings, trainees can contribute to critical thinking while analyzing and witnessing the influence of the COPC process. The cluster committee series prepares the trainee and initiates the formation of the community-professional partnership. Simultaneously, it sets the stage for the initiation, development, and implementation of a health promotion or disease prevention project.

Designed as a didactic exercise, the cluster committee brings the classroom to the community. When community members articulate priority health issues, their nominations typically have direct bearing on health status, but little to do with the medical care system. This is a powerful message for trainees.

While the professionals learn from the community by using the cluster committee series to discuss approaches to each of the five steps, community members also learn from the professionals. Because of the interactive nature of the development of a public health project, site members and community members are in a position to remain active participants in the intervention program which follows, ready for eventual institutionalization of the community-professional partnership that is the keystone of COPC.

BARRIERS THAT MAY NEED TO BE OVERCOME

With the success of COPC as a modality of practice both in and outside the United States, it is reasonable to ask, "Why hasn't this approach been adopted universally?" Some answers are found in Chapter 2, where the authors lay out the considerations one should review in deciding whether to engage in COPC. Others lie in the way health care professionals are currently educated, trained, and then paid in this country. While education and training have begun to move from within hospital walls to ambulatory and other out-of-hospital settings, simply moving the site of instruction doesn't represent training in COPC. Additionally, payment for care continues to reflect productivity, defined as number of patients seen. Until the community is viewed and understood as a patient worth caring for and paying to be cared for, the external forces required to support the type of practice that is COPC will be absent.

Significant change in the health care system will result when changing health professions education meets a changing mode of payment and organization of delivery. While there are barriers to change in education, they are not insurmountable. Recently, the external environment, represented by multiple organizations that have examined the roles, responsibilities, and competencies that health care practitioners and agencies will need in the next millennium, has shifted in support of the approach to practice that is manifested by COPC.[33] Nevertheless, barriers continue to exist:

▶ Educational institutions need to articulate a *vision* that reflects their commitment to improving community health through each leg of the stool—research, education, and service—upon which they sit. This requires strong leadership and consensus building.

▶ A reflection of educational institutions not having developed COPC curricula is that the *faculty expertise* to teach, mentor, and role model these skills and attitudes is lacking. While faculty development programs are badly needed, they should not be looked upon as an annoying, time consuming first step. Rather, if viewed as a lever for all members of an institution—students, faculty, and administrators alike—to express the vision, they can be energizing; faculty and students can then learn and practice alongside one another.

▶ *Curriculum time* needs to be dedicated to education and training in the skills needed to practice COPC. In some instances, the blocks of time already exist; the subject matter simply needs to be fitted into the COPC paradigm and be better coordinated, taught in a more cogent manner, and/or run throughout the curriculum as part of its underpinnings, i.e., continually questioning students about what any particular condition might imply *vis a vis* the community. Where these topics do not exist in the curriculum, the barrier can be daunting. Competition among departments for time and place in the schedule is intense. Change can probably be accomplished only if the institution articulates a mission to improve community health.

▶ The *community* itself may be a barrier. After years of being studied by academics, and then left to fend for themselves, communities have become cynical about working with institutions of higher education. Consequently, the trust and caring required to build an equal partnership need to be initiated, cultivated, and nurtured on a continuing basis. Communities do not tend to seek out academic institutions with which to work. Patience and honesty are essential if professionals are going to be able to develop working relationships with communities (see Example 4.1).

▶ The *external environment*, though changing, remains a barrier to teaching COPC. By and large, clinicians are paid to see patients one-on-one. Until they are compensated for working with a community to improve its health, practitioners will continue to be trained just to perform clinical duties.[34] While the primary care specialties, particularly family practice, stress the importance of understanding the link between the individual's health and the family's health, there remains little financial incentive for practitioners to understand and act on the links between an individual's health and the community's health. Nevertheless, some HMOs have begun to urge practitioners to apply elements of the theory and practice of human behavior to health promotion and disease prevention; others are considering broadening their mission from caring for enrolled populations to include contributions to the health of the communities in which they serve.[35] By conducting better outcomes studies with communities, including those defined as constituents of an HMO, the cost savings advantages of COPC can be documented. When COPC is viewed as the superior way to practice because it results in improved health at a reduced cost, the external environment will become an enabler rather than a barrier to COPC.

CONCLUSION

The skills needed for the practice of COPC as presented in this book serve as a template for a practitioner's life-long learning experiences, as well as for an organization's developing into a learning organization.[36] These skills can be used to adapt to changes in the health care system, as well as to changes that occur within communities.

The association between community health and individual health dictates that medicine cannot keep people healthy and restore them to health if they live in unhealthy communities.

The amalgamation of clinical medicine and public health, COPC principles and practice should be taught throughout a health care practitioner's educational experience.[37] That is a lifelong task, and one that often seems to run counter to external, as well as internal, pressures.

This education and training are action-oriented and grounded in community. The community must be treated respectfully as a valued partner, not simply as a laboratory for academic work. The community must act as classroom, patient, and partner. Role models are essential. Students must see the steps of COPC being carried out, and must have an opportunity to be a part of the action. This means that in many instances, faculty development programs will be essential elements of education in COPC. The COPC process and philosophy that students must understand is not simply a health promotion or disease prevention project, but rather a never ending process that spawns these projects. Education and training in COPC must be evaluated continually, with application of the short feedback loop so that programs are improved continuously.

Teaching and learning the skills and attitudes necessary for COPC practice is an energizing, broadening experience. Those who engage in this endeavor and practice these skills bring a new and deeper understanding to clinical practice. Clinical and public health skills merge, and thus COPC provides the blueprint for practice into the 21st Century.

REFERENCES

1. Cashman S, Fulmer H, Staples L. Community health: beyond care for individuals. *Social Policy.* 1994;52-62.
2. Salmon M, Viadro C. Objectives for the nation: a national agenda for nursing education, research, and practice. *Nursing Outlook.* 1989;37:110-111.
3. Stoto M. Sharing responsibility for the public's health: a new perspective from the Institute of Medicine. *J Public Health Management Practice.* 1997;3:22-34.
4. Wray J. Undergraduate and graduate education in community medicine. In: Lathem W, Newbery A, eds. *Community Medicine.* New York, NY: Appleton-Century-Crofts; 1970.
5. Kenyon V, Smith E, Hefty L, Bell M, McNeil J, Martaus T. Clinical competencies for community health nursing. *Public Health Nurs.* 1990;7:33-39.
6. Shoultz J, Hatcher P, Hurrell M. Growing edges of a new paradigm: the future of nursing in the health of the nation. *Nurs Outlook.* 1992;40:57-61.
7. Smilkstein G. Designing a curriculum for training community-responsive physicians. *J of Health Care for the Poor and Underserved.* 1990;1:237-242.
8. Klevens M, Cashman S, Margules A, Fulmer H. Transforming a neighborhood health center into a community-oriented primary care practice. *Am J Prev Med.* 1992;8:62-65.
9. Havens B, Stevens R. A continuing education model for community health nursing practice. *J Community Health Nurs.* 1990;7:123-130.
10. Kurtzman C, Block L. Preparation of nurses for community orientation in primary health care in Israel. *Israel JMed Sciences.* 1983;19:768-770.
11. Deuschle K, Fulmer H. Community medicine: a new department at the University of Kentucky. *J Med Educ.* 1962;37:434-445.
12. Fulmer H. Teaching community medicine in Kentucky. *Harvard School of Public Health Alumni Bulletin.* 1994;21:2-6.
13. Burke W, Eckhert L, Hays C, Mansell E, Deuschle K, Fulmer H. An evaluation of the undergraduate medical curriculum: the Kentucky experiment in community medicine. *JAMA.* 1979;24:2726-2730.
14. Institute of Medicine, Committee for the Study of the Future of Public Health. *The Future of Public Health.* Washington, DC: National Academy Press; 1988.
15. Deuschle K, Fulmer H, McNamara M, Tapp J. The Kentucky experiment in community medicine. *Milbank Memorial Fund Quarterly.* 1966;XLIV:9-21.
16. Hays C, Burke W, Mansell E, Fulmer H. The community as pre-clinical classroom: experience with a first year clerkship. *J Med Educ.* 1980;55:602-609.
17. Snadden D, Mowat D. Community-based curriculum development: what does it really mean? *Med Teacher.* 1995;17:297-306.
18. Smith D, Anderson R. Community-responsive medicine: a call for a new academic discipline. *J of Health Care for the Poor and Underserved.* 1990;1:219-228.
19. Anderson R, Boumboulian P. Comprehensive community health programs: a new look at an old approach. In: Korn, McLaughlin, Osterweis, eds. *Academic Health Centers in the Managed Care Environment.* Washington, DC: Association of Academic Health Centers; 1995.
20. Anderson R. Integrating community-responsive medicine into the urban safety-net hospital. In: Rogers R, Ginzberg E, eds. *The Metropolitan Academic Medical Center.* Boulder, Colo: Westview Press; 1995.
21. Fulmer H. *Preventive Medicine in Every Specialty:* Presentation to American Public Health Association, Los Angeles, Calif, October 1978.
22. Anderson A. Public health content in nursing curricula. *Nurs Outlook.* 1989;37:233-235.
23. Lane D, Ross V. The importance of defining physicians' competencies: lessons from preventive medicine. *Acad Med.* 1994;69(pt 12):972-74.

24. Competencies and performance indicators for preventive medicine residents. Washington, DC: American College of Preventive Medicine; 1993.
25. Sorensen A, Bialek R, eds. *The Public Health Faculty/Agency Forum: Linking Graduate Education and Practice*. Gainesville: Florida University Press; 1993.
26. Shugars D, O'Neill E, Bader J, eds. *Healthy America: Practitioners for 2005, An Agenda for Action for US Health Professional Schools*. Durham, NC: The Pew Health Professions Commission; 1991.
27. *The Public Health Workforce: An Agenda for the 21st Century*. Public Health Service, USDHHS; 1997.
28. Cashman S, Fulmer H, Aaberg A, Staples L. Public health nursing: a model for the 21st century. *Amer J Public Health*. 1994;84:1694-95.
29. Gardner J. *Building Community*. Washington, DC: Independent Sector; 1991.
30. Bradley B. America's challenge: revitalizing our national community. *National Civic Review*. 1995;84:94-100.
31. Thomas C, Cashman S, Fulmer H. The cluster committee: setting the stage for community-responsive care. *Am J Prev Med*. 11(pt 1):9-18.1995.
32. Thomas C, Cashman S, Fulmer H. The cluster committee: setting the stage for community-responsive health care. *Acad Med*.1994:130.
33. Recommendations of the Initiative Task Force. *The Medicine/Public Health Initiative*. Chicago, Ill: National Congress; March 1996.
34. Fulmer H, Cashman S. Community-responsive care: a new paradigm. *The Bulletin: American Association of Public Health Physicians*. 1993;39.
35. Showstack J et al. Health of the public: the private sector challenge. *JAMA*. 1996;276: 1071-1074.
36. Senge P. The leader's new work. *Sloan Management Review*.1990;7-22.
37. Fulmer H. COPC residency and fellowship training: a necessary link towards a 21st century health care system that is community responsive. *COPaCetic Newsletter*. Cleveland, Ohio: Case Western Reserve University. Autumn 1994.

APPENDIX 1.1
COPC NATIONAL RURAL DEMONSTRATION PROJECT SITES
AND PARTICIPANTS

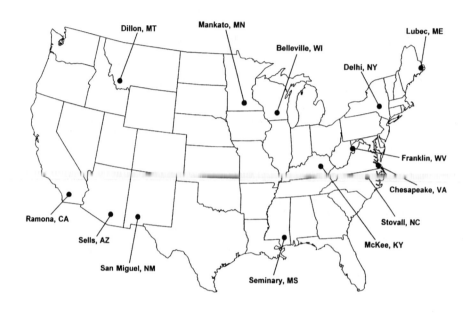

COPC NATIONAL RURAL DEMONSTRATION
PROJECT PARTICIPANTS
1988-1991

NATIONAL RURAL HEALTH ASSOCIATION
Robert Van Hook
Gary Kukulka

**HOSPITAL RESEARCH AND
EDUCATIONAL TRUST**
Richard Bogue
John Lowe

**UNIVERSITY OF NEW MEXICO
TECHNICAL CONSULTATION TEAM**
Thomas Becker
Clark Hansbarger
Martin Hickey
Norton Kalishman
Martin Kantrowitz
Laurie Kastelic
Arthur Kaufman

Cheri Koinis
Richard Kozoll
Robert Rhyne
Barbara Sheline
Betty Skipper
Christopher Urbina
Ronald Voorhees
Nina Wallerstein
Sharon Wayne
William Wiese

TOHONO O'ODHAM HEALTH DEPARTMENT
SELLS, ARIZ
Paul Fuhrmeister
Beverly Hackenberg
Robert Hackenberg
Robert Livingstone
Rosemary Lopez
Ron Rust

NORTH COUNTY HEALTH SERVICES
RAMONA, CALIF
Johanna Aiken
Betty Dodds
Janice Fearn
Charlene Hasper
James Hutzley
Diana Lacey
Sylvia Micik
Chris Walker
Janice Yuwiler

HEALTH HELP, INC.
MCKEE, KY
David Greene
Ted Kay
Angel Rubio
Susan Sweitzer

REGIONAL MEDICAL CENTER AT LUBEC
LUBEC, ME
Cathy Cook
Liz Crocker
Jane Donnell
Marilyn Hughes
Irene McMahan
Kenneth Schmidt
Ben Thompson

WELLNESS CENTER OF MINNESOTA
MANKATO, MINN
Anne Ganey
Sandy Gundlach
Linda Hachfeld
John Lester
William Manahan

SOUTHEAST MISSISSIPPI
RURAL HEALTH INITIATIVE
SEMINARY, MISS
Co-Sandra Barnes
Lynn Hartwig
Stephen Lambert
Kaye Ray
Pamela Rodgers
Lynn Sanford

BARRETT MEMORIAL HOSPITAL
DILLON, MONT
Jean Berna
Sue Hansen
Ruth Haugland
Katherine Buckley-Patton
Timothy Visscher
Vance Fager
Judith Wilson

LA CLINICA DE FAMILIA, INC.
SAN MIGUEL, NM
Berta Contreras
Frank Crespin
Judy Ingram
Mary Sanchez-Bane
Martha Liefeld

O'CONNOR DIVISION/
M.I. BASSETT HOSPITAL
DELHI, NY
Ron Coffey
Marthe Gold
Jane Hamilton
Harriet Hanoshman
Linda Haynes
Judy Macek
Frank Silagy

STOVALL MEDICAL CLINIC
STOVALL, NC
Marilyn Howard
Jim Johnson
Kathy Johnson
Jenny Koinis
Thomas Koinis

CHESAPEAKE HEALTH DEPARTMENT
CHESAPEAKE, VA
Tsegaw Lemlem
Janet Morgan
Nancy Welch
David West

BELLEVILLE FAMILY MEDICINE CLINIC
BELLEVILLE, WIS
Marma McIntee
Richard Roberts

PENDLETON COMMUNITY CARE
FRANKLIN, WVA
David Cockley
Thomas Hull
Debbie Kimble
King Seegar
Henry Taylor

NATIONAL COPC ADVISORY COMMITTEE
Jacquelyn Admire
Dan Doyle
Diane Howard
John Lowe
Craig Robinson
James Bernstein
Kevin Fickenscher
Richard Kozoll
Paul Nutting
James Schuman
Donald Weaver
Vic Cocowitch
David Garr
Joyce Lashoff
Myrna Pickard
Howard Smith

UNIVERSITY OF MINNESOTA
Jon Christianson
Ira Moscovice

ADDITIONAL CONTRIBUTORS
Eugenia Eng
Tom Ricketts

APPENDIX 1.2
COPC OPERATIONAL MODEL:
FIVE STEPS AND THEIR CORRESPONDING STAGES
(modified and adapted from Nutting - IOM COPC Operational Model)

Step 1: Defining and Characterizing the Community

Stage 0:   No effort has been made to define or characterize a community beyond the active users of the practice.

Stage I: There is no enumeration of the individuals who constitute the community. The community is characterized by extrapolation from large area census data.

Stage II: There is no enumeration of the community, but it is characterized through the use of secondary data that correspond closely to the target community.

Stage III: The community can be enumerated and is actively characterized through the use of a database that includes all members of the community and describes its demography and socioeconomic status. (Often such a data system is constructed over time from the active users of services and approximates the community closely, e.g., at or above 90 percent coverage of the community.)

Stage IV: Systematic efforts ensure a current and complete enumeration of all individuals in the community, including pertinent demographic and socioeconomic data. For each individual, information exists that facilitates targeted outreach, e.g., address, telephone number, etc.

Step 2: Involving the Community

Stage 0:   No effort is made to organize community participation or to get community input.

Stage I: The importance of community involvement is recognized, but community outreach efforts are limited and participation is superficial.

Stage II: Systematic efforts are made to invite the community to participate in and be oriented to the COPC process. Although broad-based community input is encouraged, only a few well recognized community leaders are involved.

Stage III: The community is organized and participates in the process but is not perceived as an equal partner by either the professionals or itself.

Stage IV: Extensive and formal ongoing outreach occurs. Community members, recognized leaders, and grassroots citizens participate in all aspects of the COPC process. The community members and the professionals view each other as valued partners.

Step 3: Identifying Community Health Problems

Stage 0:   No systematic efforts have been made to understand the health status or health needs of the community. Alternatively, the results from studies of the patient population are assumed to reflect the health problems in the community as a whole.

Stage I: Community health problems are identified through general consensus of the providers and/or community groups.

Stage II: Community health problems are identified by extrapolation from systematic review of secondary data, such as vital statistics, census data, large area epidemiologic data, etc.

Stage III: Community health problems are examined through the use of data sets that are specific to the community but tend to focus on single health problems or health care issues.

Stage IV: Formal mechanisms (usually but not always epidemiologic techniques) are used to identify and set priorities among a broad range of potential health problems in the community, identify their correlates and determinants, and characterize the existing patterns of health care related to the problem.

Step 4: Modifying the Health Care Program

Stage 0:   No modifications are made in the primary care program in specific response to health needs of the larger community.

Stage I: Modifications address health problems believed to exist in the community but are made more in response to a national or organization-wide initiative than in response to a particular problem identified in the community.

Stage II: Modifications address important community health problems but are chosen largely because of the availability of special resources to address that particular problem and closely follow guidelines that may not be tailored to community needs.

Stage III: Modifications in the health care program are tailored to the unique needs of the community and involve (where appropriate) both the primary care and community/public health components of the program.

Stage IV: Modifications in the program involve both primary care and community/public health components and are targeted to specific high risk or priority groups, with active efforts (e.g., outreach) made to reach those groups.

Step 5: Monitoring the Effectiveness of Program Modification

Stage 0:   Examination of program effectiveness is limited to the impact on the active users of health services.

Stage I: Program effectiveness is viewed in terms of impact on the community as a whole but is based on subjective impressions of the practitioners and/or community groups.

Stage II: Program effectiveness is estimated by extrapolation from large area data or vital statistics.

Stage III: Program effectiveness is determined by systematic examination of a data set that is specific to the community.

Stage IV: Program effectiveness is determined by techniques which are specific to the program objectives, account for differential impact among risk groups, and provide information on positive and negative impacts.

Adapted from Institute of Medicine. *Community-Oriented Primary Care: A Practical Assessment.* Washington: National Academy Press; 1982: 1:35-40.

APPENDIX 5.1
NEEDS ASSESSMENT QUESTIONNAIRE

Cross-Cultural Training Program for Health Care Providers
Survey Questionnaire

1. What is the ethnic/racial makeup of the patients/clients you serve? Please estimate the percentage for each of the population groups listed below:

ETHNIC GROUP	PERCENTAGE
Afro-American	_____
Asian/Pacific Islander	_____
Caucasian	_____
Latino	_____
Other	_____

2. What barriers have you encountered in providing care for patients/clients from ethnic or cultural groups different than your own?

_____

_____

_____

_____

3. What skill areas or issues should be addressed in a training workshop to assist health care personnel in providing culturally appropriate health care to patients/ clients from different ethnic backgrounds?

_____

_____

_____

_____

4. Do you believe such a cross-cultural training program is needed where you work?

  ❑ yes   ❑ no   ❑ unsure

Comments : _____
_____
_____
_____
_____

Have you ever participated in a similar type of training program?

  ❑ yes   ❑ no   ❑ unsure

If so, please describe and comment on its usefulness to you:
_____
_____
_____
_____
_____

5. Would you be willing to pay a fee for this type of training?
  _____

6. What is your job title? _____

7. What is your ethnic group (optional)? _____

8. Name (optional) _____

9. Agency (optional) _____

10. Other comments _____
_____
_____
_____
_____
_____

11. Each of the following are factors which can influence the quality of care provided to patients/clients from ethnic minority populations. For each item, please indicate whether or not this has been an area of difficulty for you in serving minority populations, and if so, to what extent?

Factor	no difficulty	some difficulty	much difficulty	not applicable
Verbal communication (language)	_____	_____	_____	_____
Non-verbal communication (body language)	_____	_____	_____	_____
Patient compliance with treatment	_____	_____	_____	_____
Ability to interpret patient's reporting of symptoms	_____	_____	_____	_____
Appointment keeping	_____	_____	_____	_____
Acceptance of western styles of medical treatment	_____	_____	_____	_____
Estimation of appropriate physical proximity between patient and provider	_____	_____	_____	_____
Conflict of values	_____	_____	_____	_____

Source: Overall NA, Williamson J, eds, *Community-Oriented Primary Care in Action: A Practice Manual for Primary Care Settings.* Berkeley: University of California at Berkeley, School of Public Health; 1988.

APPENDIX 5.2
ACTION PLANNING WORKSHEET

1.   Problem Identification (use operational language): _____

   _____

   _____

   _____

   _____

   _____

2.   Realistic Ideal (state in behavioral and measurable language): _____

   _____

   _____

   _____

   _____

   _____

3.   Obstacles: _____

   _____

   _____

   _____

   _____

   _____

4.   Resources: _____

   _____

   _____

_____

_____

_____

_____

_____

_____

_____

5.   Intervention Strategies: _____

_____

_____

_____

_____

_____

Action Plan

1. Statement of the Problem (What is current situation as evidenced by behaviors, events, and happenings?)

2. Realistic Ideal (What would be happening differently if things were going well? Identify population targeted, behaviors to be changed, degree of change, and target date.)

3. Obstacles (What is preventing the realistic ideal from happening right now?)

4. Resources (Who are the people, programs, organizations, $ that can help us reach our ideal?)

5. Intervention Strategies (What needs to be done to reach the realistic ideal?)

6. Evaluation (What measures will we build in to determine whether our goal is reached?)

7. Future (Next steps: next meeting date, purpose of meeting, long and short term goals, etc.)

Source: Southwest Center for Drug-Free Schools and Communities. New Mexico Community Team Training. Norman: University of Oklahoma; 1989. Used by permission.

APPENDIX 6.1
SECONDARY DATA SOURCES

1.   **US Census reports.** The US Census reports are full of information that may be useful for almost all communities in the United States. The census data are rich sources of demographic descriptors by geographic area and include data on population composition, financial resources, ethnic descriptors, as well as information on occupation and employment. US Census data are grossly underutilized by COPC researchers for characterizing communities. The challenge is to accurately describe your population using subdivisions of census areas because it can be difficult to match your community or geographic service area to the census areas. The User-Defined Areas Program (UDAP) is a census-related data source that provides summaries for geographic areas not available through the standard data products included in the 1990 Census Tabulation and Publication Program. Prospective users can order information on a UDAP form and be billed later. Among the many variables available in the census information are age, sex, number of households, income per capita, income per household, ethnicity, occupations, and other employment data.

2.   **United States vital records.** Another underutilized resource is the mortality data published annually by the federal government. Housed in most major libraries, the natality (birth) and mortality summaries provide useful information on ethnic or racial differences in mortality on a cause and age-specific basis. We have frequently used New Mexico's vital records data in identifying statewide priorities in health provision; we have also used statewide mortality data in the US vital statistics reports to support grant applications for various infectious and chronic diseases. The reports have been published for several decades for persons interested in gaining an historic perspective on mortality rates in their area or nationwide. Data include county mortality rates by cause of death, age, sex, and race, and years of potential life lost, and can be used to calculate trends.

3.   **Focused federal reports on specific health issues.** The US Department of Health and Human Services has published a series of volumes on minority health issues. These cover such topics as cardiovascular and cerebrovascular diseases, black and Hispanic health issues, and diseases and

health priorities of particular concern to American Indians/Alaska Native peoples nationwide. Although the data are not commonly broken down by community, many of these ethnic or racial-specific issues apply to COPC projects. In particular, the data can support a decision to investigate a specific problem within an ethnic or racial group.

The National Institutes of Health, through the US Department of Health and Human Services, has also published focused monographs on cancer among blacks and other minorities, including in-depth statistical profiles. Such monographs are published routinely and contain vital background information for COPC activities. In particular, the chart book series provides annual updates on topics such as the health of disadvantaged peoples.

4. State vital statistics summary. Every state publishes annual reports containing selected health statistics, which are extremely useful to assess infectious and chronic disease problems on a county- or community-wide level. In addition to information on natality and mortality, many of the state vital records reports contain incidence data on specific diseases such as cancer and certain infectious diseases. Some of these records also present analyses of years of potential life lost to specific diseases and comparisons of state or county rates with national rates. The county or city level summaries are especially helpful; in New Mexico, we use them in identifying community-related problems that are very important in one or two counties, but less problematic in the rest of the state.

Some state data are available on computerized tapes, since births and deaths are public record. Case counts by cause of death can be analyzed in terms of age-specific or race-specific rates of mortality. Since most states collect such data by city or county of residence, the tapes can be examined in reference to a specific community. Although vital records data are fraught with potential bias (symptoms, signs, and ill-defined conditions), we nonetheless have used these tapes to help guide several projects.

5. Disease registries. Some states and/or cities have disease registries which are enormously helpful. Several states and approximately a dozen cities have cancer registries, some supported by the National Cancer Institute, which calculate age-, ethnic- and sex-specific incidence rates for various cancers and commonly follow the course of disease, treatment, and survival and include data on treatment modalities. At the city, county, and even state levels, such data can be particularly important for helping to guide screening or preventive efforts. For example, cervical cancer is a particular problem among minority women in parts of the United States. The magnitude of rate differences by ethnic or racial groups can be determined from cancer registries, which also include place of residence and can therefore be used to investigate cancer rates on a county or regional basis. The caveat, of course, is that there must be enough cases (numerators) and adequately described denominators to conclude something meaningful about a rate or risk of developing a specific cancer.

Several communities also have trauma registries based on city, county, or state population that can provide important information on incidence and location of various injuries.

6.   Indian Health Service (IHS) reports. For those interested in COPC within Native American communities, the IHS publishes annual reports on disease incidence and mortality on an area-specific or tribe-specific basis. The IHS also maintains an elaborate system of outpatient and inpatient records, which can be accessed via computer on a clinic-hospital-tribe or IHS area-specific basis.

7.   County Coroner or Office of the Medical Investigator reports. Various county and state coroner systems nationwide keep impressive records on cause of death, age, race, sex, circumstances surrounding death, place of death, place of birth, and accompanying medical conditions not directly related to cause of death. Specific information on organ or organ system damage are also frequently reported for those cases undergoing post-mortem examination. We have found the statewide Office of the Medical Investigator data collection system to be an underutilized, valuable resource in helping us recognize ethnic and sex-specific differences in mortality for various causes of death.

8.   Poison and drug information centers. Most major US cities have reporting systems for poison control. A detailed data set is collected with each telephone call to a poison/drug information center. The data often include potential occupational exposures and other relevant information. For COPC projects focused specifically on poison-related injuries, such data sets are extremely valuable, not only as background for choosing COPC projects, but also for monitoring the effect of an intervention.

9.   Police and fire department reports. Most communities keep computerized records of police and fire department activities such as investigation of child and elderly abuse incidence, including information on victims and alleged perpetrators. Fire departments frequently record the numbers and types of runs made, including those for elderly victims of fall-related events. County sheriff and fire departments keep comparable records.

10. State and local health departments. State and local health departments frequently maintain detailed records of motor vehicle-related events, including accidents, injury statistics, and fatal outcomes. Reports can also include data on alcohol or drug use that may have affected injury events. Maps may outline areas of various communities that are particularly problematic in terms of traffic accidents. Such data can be very important for gauging the magnitude of various problems and evaluating subsequent interventions.

11. Statewide or local offices of epidemiology. Epidemiology offices collect and analyze data for many acute infectious and chronic diseases. Office organization varies from state to state, with some states centralizing reporting through the state health department, and other states dividing reporting differently. Epidemiology offices are very helpful in assessing or monitoring project intervention. For example, if a COPC project based on a series of adolescent health care clinics determines that specific sexually transmitted diseases are the problem priority for the clinic, changes in disease rates after intervention can be monitored through the epidemiology offices, in collaboration with the laboratories that report culture results.

12. Hospital epidemiologist. Most major hospitals employ infection control personnel who are responsible for monitoring positive culture results, both viral and bacterial, within a catchment area. Such records are useful in prioritizing various infectious diseases within a community and may prove even more useful than statewide or countywide reporting, depending on the community chosen.

13. University data. Many universities have a large data processing and/or data collection system that is specific to the state or community in which it is located. At the University of New Mexico, the UNM Data Bank curates census information, vital record data, special reports on diseases and state trends in disease incidence, economic profiles of various communities and states, and county and community population rates. The Data Bank also has such diverse data as occupational injuries and illnesses that may have occurred in the state or in a community during a given period of time.

14. Behavioral Risk Factor Surveillance System (BRFS). In 1990, 44 states and the District of Columbia participated in monthly random-digit telephone interviews of adults over 18 years of age to compile information on several major public health issues, including summaries of knowledge/attitudes/ behavior on topics such as seat belt use, hypertension, exercise, weight control, tobacco use, alcohol use, drinking and driving laws, preventive health practices, diabetes, health insurance, women's health issues, AIDS (HIV infection), injury control, and nutrition.

Many states have added data on other issues of local or statewide importance that allow examination by sex, age, ethnicity/race, and location of residence.

15. Area Resource File. The Office of Data Analysis and Management (ODAM) maintains a health resources information system for the Bureau of Health Professions (BHPr). This system, the Area Resource File System (ARFS), is designed for use by health analysts and other professionals seeking consistent, current, and compatible information on the nation's health care delivery system. It consists of four major components: the basic Area Resource File (ARF), a massive county-specific database; a State/ National Timeseries database; a microcomputer data series containing demographic, health facilities, and health professions data extracts for use on microcomputers; and internal components including detailed hospital files and over 50 detailed disciplinary support files.

The ARFS serves as a major tool for the Bureau of Health Professionals to carry out its mandated program of:

► Research and analysis of the geographic distribution (or maldistribution) of health manpower;

► Analysis of health manpower supply, utilization, requirements, costs, and related issues; and

► Development and refinement of long-range forecasts of health professions supply and requirements.

ARFS aims to provide:

► The most timely and accurate health-related data available at the county level;

► Compatible and consistent data;

► Data in a variety of forms for use by the broadest possible range of users; and

► Flexible capabilities for analysis of health-related data.

16. Miscellaneous. An enormous number of other data resources are available for use in COPC projects. For example, university or student health centers generally collect and curate the incidence and/or prevalence of the diseases they treat. Many county and state programs also collect clinic-specific or community-specific data on diseases. Medical librarians who are familiar with these more obscure data resources, including other government documents, can be valuable resources for targeting your programs.

APPENDIX 6.2
REGIONAL CENSUS OFFICES

Census information can be accessed by contacting your regional census bureau office.

Atlanta, GA	(404) 730-3833/3964 (TDD)
Boston, Mass	(617) 424-0510/0565 (TTD)
Charlotte, NC	(704) 344-6144/6548 (TDD)
Chicago, Ill	(708) 562-1740/1791 (TDD)
Dallas, Tex	(214) 640-4470/4434 (TDD)
Denver, Col	(303) 969-7750/6769 (TDD)
Detroit, Mich	(313) 259-1875/5169 (TDD)
Kansas City, Mo	(913) 551-6711/5839 (TTD)
Los Angeles, Calif	(818) 904-6339/6249 (TDD)
New York, NY	(212) 264-4730/3863 (TDD)
Philadelphia, Penn	(215) 656-7578/7550 (TDD)
Seattle, Wash	(206) 553-5835/5859 (TDD)

Regional Office Liaison .... (301) 457-2032

http://www.census.gov

APPENDIX 6.3
GEOGRAPHIC ENTITIES OF THE 1990 CENSUS

TYPE OF GEOGRAPHIC ENTITY	STATUS	NUMBER
Nation (the United States)[1]	Legal	1
Regions (of the United States)	Statistical	4
Divisions (of the United States)	Statistical	9
States and Statistically Equivalent Entities[2]	Legal	57
Counties and Statistically Equivalent Entities	Legal	3,248
County Subdivisions and Places		60,228
Minor Civil Divisions (MDCs)	Legal	30,386
Sub-MCDs	Legal	145
Census County Divisions (CCDs)	Statistical	5,581
Unorganized Territories (UTs)	Statistical	282
Other Statistically Equivalent Entities[3]	Statistical	40
Incorporated Places[4]	Legal	19,365
Consolidated Cities	Legal	6
Census Designated Places (CDPs)	Statistical	4,423
American Indian and Alaska Native Areas (AIANAs)		576
American Indian Reservations (no trust lands)	Legal	259
American Indian Entities with Trust Lands	Legal	52
Tribal Jurisdiction Statistical Areas (TJSAs)	Statistical	19
Tribal Designated Statistical Areas (TDSAs)	Statistical	17
Alaska Native Village Statistical Areas (ANVSAs)	Statistical	217
Alaska Native Regional Corporations (ANRCs)	Legal	12
Metropolitan Areas (MAs)		362
Metropolitan Statistical Areas (MSAs)	Statistical	268
Consolidated Metropolitan Statistical Areas (CMSAs)	Statistical	21
Primary Metropolitan Statistical Areas (PMSAs)	Statistical	73
Urbanized Areas (UAs)	Statistical	405
Special-Purpose Entities		404,583
Congressional Districts	Legal	435
Voting Districts (VTDs)[5]	Legal	148,872
School Districts	Administrative	15,274
Traffic Analysis Zones (TAZs)[6]	Administrative	200,000
ZIP Codes[7]	Administrative	40,000
Census Tracts and Block Numbering Areas (BNAs)		62,276
Census Tracts	Statistical	50,690
Block Numbering Areas	Statistical	11,586
Block Groups (BGs)	Statistical	229,192
Blocks	Statistical	7,017,427

1. Officially, "the United States" consists of the 50 States and the District of Columbia.
2. In addition to the 50 States and the District of Columbia (the United States), the 1990 decennial census includes American Samoa, Guam, the Northern Mariana Islands, Palau, Puerto Rico, and the Virgin Islands of the United States.
3. The 40 entities include the 40 "census subareas" in Alaska.
4. In agreement with the State of Hawaii, the Census Bureau does not recognize the city of Honolulu, which is coextensive with Honolulu County, as an incorporated place for statistical presentation purposes. Instead, the State delineates, and the Census Bureau tabulates data for, CDPs that define the separate communities within Honolulu County.
5. Include only those eligible entities participating under the provisions of Public Law 94-171.
6. The number of Traffic Analysis Zones, for which the Census Bureau tabulated data from the 1990 census, is an estimated value.
7. The number of ZIP Codes is an estimated value.

APPENDIX 6.4
THE CENSUS BUREAU'S MOST COMMONLY USED STATISTICAL ENTITIES

Region and Division[1] Combination of States.

Metropolitan Area (MA)[1] One or more contiguous counties (cities and towns in New England) that are socially and economically integrated with a large densely settled population core.

Urbanized Area (UA) A continuously built-up area with a population of 50,000 or more.

Census County Division (CCD) A subdivision of a county that serves as the statistical equivalent of an MCD in 21 States where MCDs either do not exist or are not appropriate for decennial census data-reporting purposes.

Unorganized Territory (UT) A subdivision of a county that is the statistical equivalent of an MCD for decennial census data-reporting purposes in those MCD States that have counties with part or all of their area not in any MCD.

Census Designated Place (CDP) A densely settled population concentration which has a name and community identity but is not part of any incorporated place.

Census Tract A statistical subdivision of selected counties—established by a local committee of data users—that is a relatively stable basis for tabulating decennial census data. Secondarily, it serves as a framework for assigning census block numbers. *Tabulated parts* occur where a county subdivision or place boundary divides a census tract.

Block Numbering Area (BNA) A statistical subdivision of counties without census tracts, serving as a framework for assigning census block numbers and for tabulating decennial census data. *Tabulated parts* occur where a county subdivision or place boundary divides a BNA.

Block Group (BG) A grouping of census blocks having the same first digit in their identifying number within a census tract or BNA. *Tabulated parts* occur where a county subdivision or place boundary divides a BG.

Census Block The smallest Census Bureau geographic entity; it generally is an area bounded by streets, streams, and the boundaries of legal and statistical entities.

1. The Census Bureau tabulates data for regions, divisions, and MAs in its data presentations for almost all censuses and sample surveys. It tabulates data for other kinds of statistical entities only in its data presentations for the decennial census of population and housing, and selectively for other censuses and sample surveys.

APPENDIX 8.1
RANDOM NUMBER TABLE AND EXAMPLES

					C O L U M N							
ROW	1	2	3	4	5	6	7	8	9	10	11	12
01	9001	1532	2504	8207	4444	6013	9934	6116	5095	3904	2002	6628
02	3288	6153	6057	6725	2208	9472	6301	4585	5411	6975	6833	4581
03	2050	1988	8018	6838	9805	7625	6320	6005	9649	4536	6346	6176
04	8636	2448	4801	6913	5667	9074	8875	1517	9079	4390	3817	1259
05	8777	6193	0616	3028	6907	8584	3540	3765	5465	5604	8544	5366
06	9564	6298	2607	2557	4391	1233	5206	6095	6005	5053	9444	1796
07	6558	5980	7107	7065	8380	1989	0675	3071	1410	3619	9031	1666
08	0650	1745	6770	4410	7228	4366	6421	6438	1536	2890	6718	3603
09	4161	8203	1356	5926	8737	0034	8828	7744	6562	4067	7213	2164
10	8129	4651	0771	5981	0510	7933	6236	7737	7802	3341	3485	4254
11	4208	2289	4923	2756	3752	7158	4675	2620	6841	5943	3549	3433
12	0063	7930	4825	3176	2789	8745	0448	3639	9595	0541	8428	1863
13	4456	5734	0837	5999	5633	3933	6902	4157	1508	9784	6725	5584
14	0989	7628	8806	6755	6770	5625	2380	4109	4361	5609	1752	9207
15	9354	3506	1862	6033	5137	1387	0707	3100	7688	7601	7278	1023
16	6523	7320	5448	2402	7592	1405	6359	0346	2448	7352	8202	5465
17	0063	8161	4025	1790	7907	9084	2760	4440	8781	4550	9263	0201
18	0029	1648	6754	8361	0749	0666	1652	1785	5526	7330	1393	3196
19	1337	6988	9313	0339	7604	2571	1395	3338	6993	7734	8678	4875
20	4617	5777	3987	1419	2396	8003	2565	3640	8068	1045	2086	5790
21	0839	0700	5708	8093	8859	3029	7872	0750	2025	0897	2552	2647
22	8401	0219	1868	8456	6014	8374	1408	8575	8170	8573	0345	8762
23	4966	7813	4551	7056	2249	2196	5971	4468	9582	3662	8385	2422
24	0567	7439	2517	5193	1853	3769	2600	4751	7445	2904	4050	2786
25	4161	5999	4354	3601	2509	5209	2064	4857	6955	3440	3195	9114

This is a portion of a random number table. Numbers have been put in columns to make it easier to read the table, but the rows and columns have no meaning. You can start anywhere in the table and go up or down; every number you come across has an equally likely chance as any other number to be in that position.

Example 1: RANDOM ASSIGNMENT of four people to comparison group and four people to intervention group. Even numbers can be used to indicate assignment to the comparison group, while odd numbers can be used to indicate assignment to the intervention group. Close your eyes and point to the table to pick a random starting point. If you pick row 7 and column 6, the next 6 random numbers are 1, 9, 8, 9, 0, 6, 7, and 5. That means that the assignment of people to groups will be:

> Person 1: .... Intervention
> Person 2: .... Intervention
> Person 3: .... Comparison
> Person 4: .... Intervention
> Person 5: .... Comparison
> Person 6: .... Comparison
> Person 7: .... Intervention
> Person 8: .... Comparison

Person 8 is assigned to the comparison group even though the random number is an odd number because there are already four people assigned to the intervention group.

Example 2: SYSTEMATIC SAMPLE WITH A RANDOM START for choosing a 5% sample of medical charts. Since 5% is 1/20th of the total number of charts, you need to choose a random number between 1 and 20. Assume that you randomly start at row 4 and column 11. The first two numbers are 38, a number that is not between 1 and 20. The next two numbers are 17. You would then choose chart 17 and every 20th chart after that (i.e., 37, 57, 77, etc.)

Example 3: RANDOM DIGIT DIALING to sample a geographic area assumed to have the same three-number telephone prefix. Close your eyes and point to a place on the table. If you pick row 14 and column 2, each four digit number placed with the known prefix is a random local phone number. Reading across from row 14, column 2, the next five phone numbers would be (assuming a 272- prefix) 272-7628, 272-8806, 272-6755, 272-6770, and 272-5625. Exclude businesses and other non-residential phone numbers, and keep going until you reach the desired number of telephone respondents.

APPENDIX 8.2
SAMPLE SIZE GRAPHS

Graph 1: Alpha = .05; Power = .70

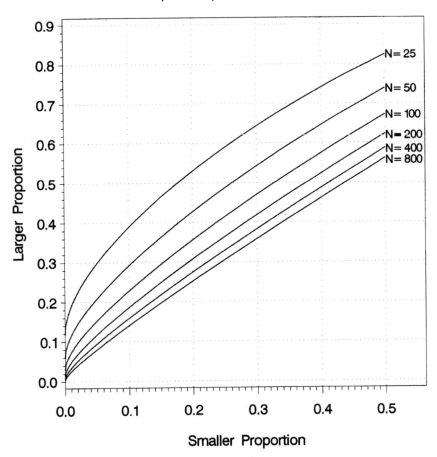

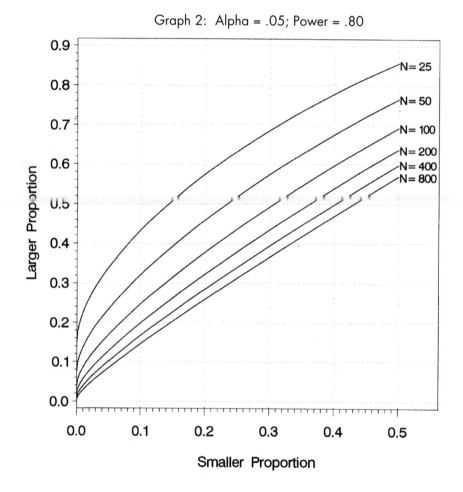

Graph 2: Alpha = .05; Power = .80

Graph 3: Alpha = .05; Power = .90

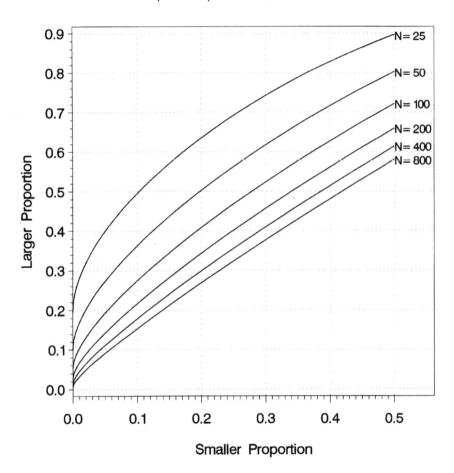

INDEX